WILLIAM SEARS, M.D., and MARTHA SEARS, R.N., are the pediatrics experts to whom American parents are increasingly turning for advice and information on all aspects of pregnancy, birth, childcare, and family nutrition. Dr. Sears was trained at Harvard Medical School's Children's Hospital and Toronto's Hospital for Sick Children, the largest children's hospital in the world. He has practiced pediatrics for nearly thirty years and currently serves as a medical and parenting consultant to *Baby Talk* and *Parenting* magazines. Martha Sears is a registered nurse, certified childbirth educator, and breastfeeding consultant. The Searses are the parents of eight children.

More information about the Searses can be found at www.SearsParenting.com and www.AskDrSears.com.

SEARS PARENTING LIBRARY

The Pregnancy Book
The Baby Book
The Birth Book
The Breastfeeding Book
The Fussy Baby Book
The Discipline Book
The Family Nutrition Book
The A.D.D. Book
The Attachment Parenting Book

PARENTING.COM FAQ BOOKS

The First Three Months
How to Get Your Baby to Sleep
Keeping Your Baby Healthy
Feeding the Picky Eater

SEARS CHILDREN'S LIBRARY

Baby on the Way
What Baby Needs

The First Three Months

America's Foremost Baby and
Childcare Experts Answer the Most
Frequently Asked Questions

William Sears, M.D., and Martha Sears, R.N.

Little, Brown and Company
BOSTON | NEW YORK | LONDON

FIRST EDITION

The information herein is not intended to replace the services of trained health professionals. You are advised to consult with your child's health-care professional with regard to matters relating to your child's health, and in particular matters that may require diagnosis or medical attention.

Library of Congress Cataloging-in-Publication Data

Sears, William, M.D.
 The first three months / by William Sears and Martha Sears — 1st ed.
  p. cm.
 Includes index.
 ISBN 0-316-77668-8
 1. Infants — Care. 2. Child care. I. Sears, Martha. II. Title.
RJ61.S44186 2001
649'.122 — dc21   00-045646

10 9 8 7 6 5 4 3 2 1

Book design and text composition by L&G McRee

Printed in the United States of America

Introduction

You are now the parents of a beautiful new baby! While it's hard to focus on the reality of child rearing in the midst of nestling that newborn, we've found many new parents and parents-to-be are often totally unprepared for what lies ahead when baby arrives.

During your pregnancy you may have buried yourselves in baby books or spent hours surfing the latest parenting sites on the Internet. Still, no matter how much research you've done, if you're like most parents-to-be, you have no idea how this precious baby will turn your once-organized, in-control lives totally upside down.

The first weeks at home are a period we call "nesting in"—a time to learn to fit together as a family. It's important to know ahead of time you will be hit with some big transitions during this time. In fact, most women undergo more turmoil in the first month after the birth of their baby than they do at any other time in their life. Your hormones are flip-flopping, your body and mind are changing, your once-stable marriage is suddenly transformed, and, if you have other children, they are undergoing adjustments as well.

New dads may have even more difficulty adapting to life with a new baby than moms do. Most dads have two new jobs at home now: not only sharing in the care of the newborn but also helping in the recuperation of the mother. In our experience, many fathers are uncomfortable handling tiny babies and equally disconcerted attending to a postpartum mother whose hormonal changes may prevent her from being the most pleasant company for a while.

As you read the questions and answers in this book, take comfort in the fact that millions of moms and dads have crossed the transition into parenthood before you— and made it! Learn from their situations to keep your first postpartum weeks joyful instead of jolting as you focus on forging ties with your newborn and each other.

With this in mind, we present the most frequently asked questions from new parents who have come before you and have felt the insecurity, exhaustion, and difficulty in adjustment that you may feel. Life with a new baby may be a time of transition, but if you prepare for this unsettling but exhilarating period, you can better enjoy yourselves and your new child.

WILLIAM SEARS, M.D., and MARTHA SEARS, R.N.

The First Three
Months

Preparing for Baby's Arrival

Q *I'm one month from delivery and cannot wait to enjoy my newborn! Still, I'm unsure about what sort of equipment I am going to need for her. What do you suggest?*

A We often refer to new parents today as the "stuff generation." When our children come to visit with our grandchildren and unload the car, we remark, "How on Earth could we have raised eight children without so much stuff?" Basically, babies need touch and human relationships more than things. But part of the fun of having a baby is designing and equipping the nursery and buying for baby. Here are some tips!

- *Buy the basics.* Purchase only what you will need for the first couple of weeks. As soon as baby arrives, so do the gifts. Besides the gifts that come pouring in at baby showers, expect grandparents to splurge.
- *Plan now—buy later.* Make a list of items you need and items you want. Check off the items that you are given or are able to borrow and purchase the rest as the need arises.
- *Beg and borrow.* Don't expect to fund this operation by yourself. You'll have lots of backers. Borrow furniture that has a short-lived use, such as a crib.
- *Choose quick-access clothing.* Keep in mind that you will be dressing a moving target that flaps around like a fish

out of water. When admiring an irresistible outfit, imagine dressing your baby. Does it give you easy access to the diaper area? Is the head opening roomy enough? Does it contain neck snaps to make it easy to slip on?

One indispensable baby item you will need is a baby sling. Wearing your baby around the house in a sling-type carrier not only makes life easier for you but also does good things for baby. Let friends and relatives know that top on your wish list is a sling-type baby carrier.

Another major consideration in buying for baby is where baby is going to sleep. Since there are several options, you may want to wait a while before splurging on an expensive crib. If you plan on sleeping with your baby in your bed at least for the first few months, you may not need a crib at all. A very popular item that is a compromise between having your baby in your bed and letting baby sleep alone in a crib is a bedside co-sleeper—a criblike infant bed that safely attaches to the side of your bed. With a co-sleeper, baby has her own space and you have yours, yet she is within arm's reach for close touch and nursing. (See Resources for Childcare Products and Information, page 129.) Other basic items you will need are:

- ☐ Three to four terry-cloth sleepers
- ☐ Three pairs of booties or socks
- ☐ Two receiving blankets
- ☐ Three undershirts
- ☐ Three lightweight tops (sacques and/or gowns)
- ☐ Diapering equipment: pail, diaper-rash cream
- ☐ Breastfeeding supplies: three nursing bras, breast pads, nursing blouses and dresses, nursing pillow
- ☐ If bottlefeeding: four 4-ounce bottles, four nipples,

measuring pitchers, spoons, utensils for washing bottles (tongs, bottle brush, sterilizing pot)

☐ Bedding supplies: two rubber-backed waterproof pads, three crib or bassinet sheets, three flannel or linen covers, bassinet blankets, weight-appropriate to the season

☐ Bathing supplies: two soft washcloths, two terry-cloth towels with hoods, mild soap and shampoo, baby bathtub

☐ Toiletries and medical supplies: mild laundry soap, petroleum jelly, rectal thermometer, baby nail clippers, antiseptic for cord care, nasal aspirator for cleaning out baby's nose, antibacterial ointment, cotton balls and swabs, vaporizer

☐ Nursery furnishings: changing table, changing-table cover and pads, rocking chair with footstool, storage chest for clothing

☐ On-the-go accessories: car seat, car-seat cover, car-seat headrest, diaper bag

✑

Sling Babies

Q *All my sister-in-law talks about is her special "sling baby." Why is carrying a baby in a sling so beneficial anyway?*

A I would like to introduce you to a style of parenting that will bring out the best in your baby and yourself. During my nearly thirty years as a pediatrician, I've often heard parents in our practice say, "As long as I carry my

baby, she's content." After years of watching a whole
parade of babywearers, we dubbed these thriving infants
"sling babies."

Many kids ago, we noticed that the more we carried our
own babies, the less they cried. I remember one day when
Martha fashioned a sling out of material from an old bed-
sheet. She said, "I really enjoy wearing Matthew. The sling
is like a piece of clothing. I put it on in the morning and
take it off in the evening."

Hence, the term babywearing was born in the Sears
household, and we developed the BabySling.® As millions
have discovered, wearing infants in a soft carrier does
good things for babies and makes life easier for Mom and
Dad. Here's why:

- *Sling babies cry less.* Parents of fussy babies who try
  babywearing report that their babies seem to forget to
  fuss. In 1986 a team of researchers in Montreal conduct-
  ed a study of ninety-nine mother-infant pairs, half of
  which were asked to carry their babies in their arms or in
  a carrier for at least three extra hours a day. After six
  weeks, the infants who received supplemental carrying
  cried and fussed 43 percent less than the noncarried
  group.
- *Sling babies learn more.* If infants spend less time crying
  and fussing, what do they do with their free time? They
  learn! Sling babies do not sleep a lot more but actually
  show increased awake contentment time called quiet
  alertness. This is the behavioral state in which an infant is
  most content and best able to interact with the environment. It may be called the optimal state of learning for a
  baby. Researchers have also reported that carried babies
  show enhanced visual and auditory alertness. A sling
  baby learns a great deal in the arms of a busy caregiver.

- *Sling babies are more organized.* It's easier to understand the benefits of babywearing when you think of a baby's gestation period as eighteen months—nine months inside the womb and at least nine more months outside the womb. The womb environment regulates baby's systems automatically. Birth temporarily disrupts this organization. The more quickly, however, baby gets outside help with organizing his systems, the more easily he adapts to the puzzle of life outside the womb. By extending the womb experience, the babywearing mother or father provides an external regulating system that balances the irregular and disorganized tendencies of the baby. Picture how these regulating systems work. Mother's rhythmic walk, for example, which baby has been feeling for nine months, reminds baby of the womb experience. This familiar rhythm, imprinted on baby's mind in the womb, now reappears in the "outside womb" and calms baby. Mother's heartbeat, beautifully regular and familiar, reminds baby of the sounds of the womb as baby places her ear against her mother's chest.
- *Sling babies are easier to breastfeed.* Babywearing allows breastfeeding "on the move," so that busy mothers can nurture their babies with the best nutrition while continuing their active lifestyles.
- *Sling babies are easier to take out.* For a baby, home is where the mother is. If you're a few weeks postpartum and you're starting to go stir crazy or feeling homebound, there's nothing in the mother-infant contract that says you have to stay home and become a recluse after you have a baby. Yet most new mothers do not feel ready to leave their babies and go out. Babywearing allows you to "have your baby and take her with you."
- *Sling babies are easier to travel with.* Busy parents throughout the world are on the go, and babywearing

makes traveling easier. During travel, babies are constantly required to make the transition from one activity
to another. Babywearing makes movement easier. While
you are standing in line at the airport, a baby worn is
safe, secure, and happy. Wearing your baby in a sling
provides a protective environment for baby when you
are shopping or sightseeing in crowds.

Babywearing tip for working moms: One way to be sure
your baby receives a lot of interaction in your absence and
is not put in the crib and left unattended is to insist that
your caregiver wear your baby at least two hours a day.
Show and tell: Show her how to wear your baby, and tell
her all about the benefits of babywearing.

✑

Baby Bonding Is Best
When You Room-In

Q *Where is the best place for my baby in the hospital?
Should I request that he stay in my room, or is he safer in
the nursery?*

A Unless a medical complication prevents it, the best
place for baby is next to Mommy. If you or baby are medically unable to room-in together, let the baby's dad or
another caring adult give baby a great deal of touch. Once
you and baby are reunited, do catch-up bonding.

Rooming-in is the option we encourage most mothers and babies to enjoy. Full rooming-in allows you to exercise your mothering instincts when the hormones in your body are programmed for it. (All hospitals that plan on staying in the "baby business" now also encourage rooming-in as it saves them dollars spent on nursing staff.) In our experience—and that of others who study newborns—a mother and baby who fully room-in enjoy the following benefits:

- Full rooming-in changes the caregiving mind-set of the attending personnel. They focus their attention and care on the mother, who is then more comfortable and able to focus on her baby.
- Rooming-in newborns cry less and more readily organize their sleep-wake cycles.
- Babies in a large nursery are sometimes soothed by tape recordings of a human heartbeat or music. Rather than being soothed electronically, the baby who is rooming-in with the mother is soothed by real and familiar sounds, which work better.
- Mother has fewer breastfeeding problems. Her milk appears sooner, and baby seems more satisfied.
- Rooming-in babies get less jaundiced, probably because they get more milk.
- A rooming-in mother usually gets more rest because she experiences less separation anxiety. In the first few days newborns sleep most of the time anyway. It is a myth that mothers of nursery-reared babies get more rest.
- Rooming-in mothers, in our experience, have a lower incidence of postpartum depression.
- Rooming-in is especially helpful for women who have difficulty jumping right into mothering.

Consider the two options:

Rooming-In Scenario

One day while making rounds I visited Jan, a new mother, only to find her sad. "What's wrong?" I inquired.

"All those gushy feelings I'm supposed to have about my baby—well, I don't have any," Jan confided. "In fact, I'm nervous, tense, and don't know what to do."

I encouraged Jan, saying, "Love at first sight doesn't happen to every couple, in courting or in parenting. For some mother-infant pairs, love is a slow and gradual process. Don't worry; your baby will help you. But you have to set the conditions that allow the mother-infant care system to click in." And I went on to explain.

All babies are born with a group of special qualities called attachment-promoting behaviors. These are features and behaviors designed to alert the caregiver to the baby's presence and draw the caregiver toward baby like a magnet. These features are the roundness of baby's eyes, cheeks, and body; the softness of the skin; the relative bigness of baby's eyes; the penetrating gaze; the incredible newborn scent; and, perhaps most important of all, baby's early language—the cries and precrying noises.

Here's how the early mother-infant communication system works. The opening sounds of baby's cry activate a mother's emotions. This is physical as well as psychological. Upon hearing her baby cry, a mother experiences an increased flow of blood to her breasts, accompanied by the biological urge to pick up and nurse her baby. This is one of the strongest examples of how the signals of the baby trigger a physiological response in the mother. There is no other signal in the world that sets off such intense responses in a mother as her baby's cry.

Picture what happens when babies and mothers room-in together. Baby begins to cry. Because the mother is right there and physically attuned to baby, she immediately picks up and feeds her infant. Baby stops crying. When baby again awakens, squirms, grimaces, and then cries, Mother responds in the same manner. The next time, the mother notices her baby's *precrying* cues. When baby awakens, squirms, and grimaces, Mother picks up and feeds baby *before* he has to cry. She has learned to read her baby's signals and to respond appropriately. After rehearsing this dialogue many times during the hospital stay, mother and baby are working as a team. Baby learns to cue better; Mother learns to respond better. As the attachment-promoting cries elicit a hormonal response in the mother, her milk-ejection reflex functions smoothly, and mother and infant are in harmony.

Baby-in-a-Plastic-Box Scenario

Now contrast the rooming-in scene above with that of an infant cared for in the hospital nursery. Picture this new-born infant lying in a plastic box. He awakens hungry and cries, along with twenty other hungry babies in plastic boxes who have by now all managed to awaken one another. A kind and caring nurse hears the cries and responds as soon as time permits. But she has no biological attachment to this baby, no inner programming tuned to this particular newborn, nor do her hormones change when baby cries. The crying, hungry baby is taken to his mother in due time. The problem is that baby's cry has two phases. The early sounds of the cry have an attachment-promoting quality, whereas the later sounds of the unattended cry are more disturbing to listen to and may actually promote avoidance on the part of the caregiver.

The mother who missed the opening scene in this

drama because she was not present when her baby started
to cry is nonetheless expected to give a nurturing response
to her baby some minutes later. But by the time the nursery-reared baby is presented to the mother, the infant has
either given up and gone back to sleep (withdrawal from
pain) or greets the mother with even more intense and
upsetting wails. The mother hears only the cries that are
more likely to elicit agitated concern rather than tender-
ness. Even though she has a comforting breast to offer
baby, she may be so tied up in knots that her milk won't
eject, and baby cries even harder. As she grows to doubt
her ability to comfort her baby, the infant may wind up
spending *more* time in the nursery, where, she feels, the
"experts" can better care for him. This separation leads to
more missed cues and breaks in the attachment between
mother and baby, and they go home from the hospital without knowing each other.

When I was in charge of a university hospital newborn
unit, we had a saying: "Nursery-reared babies cry *harder;*
rooming-in babies cry *better.*" By spending time together
and rehearsing the cue-response dialogue, baby and mother learn to fit together well—and to bring out the best in
each other.

ℒ

Single Mothers and Newborns

Q   *I'm going to have a baby next month on my own,
without a husband or partner. Is there any special advice
that you have for a single woman giving birth?*

A While you may be delivering your baby without the help of a husband or partner, you don't need to deliver your baby on your own. You may have heard the myth that partners are "labor coaches." Although that term sounds official, in reality men coach sports, not laboring women!

Both Lamaze and Bradley have emphasized the role of the father as labor coach. But few men are comfortable with this role, and few women find their mate's play-by-play strategizing helpful. The fact that there will not be a significant male supporting you at your birth should not detract from your joy of birthing, and it may even help you have an easier birth. Some men do not handle birth well and regard the normal birth scene as a problem—they want to rush and fix it.

You may want to consider having professional labor support, and usually women make better labor support persons than do men. Both studies and common sense show that the probability of having a satisfying birth and a healthy baby is increased by the presence of someone who provides accurate information and support and empowers a woman to work with her body and make wise birthing choices. A professional labor assistant (PLA) really shines in crisis moments during delivery, especially if there is an unanticipated complication or sudden change in birth plans, requiring decisions to be made about technology or surgery. During these situations, a laboring woman often does not have a clear enough mind to understand her options completely. The PLA acts as her advocate or a go-between with the medical staff, often interpreting the medical information for her so that she can more easily understand and be part of the decision.

The PLA is a woman and probably a mother herself. She brings the relaxed, natural approach of the midwife to a traditional hospital birth. Though a friend can certainly be a labor support person, mothers typically have the best results when they hire a PLA, also called a labor support doula or a monitrice. In addition to providing comfort and companionship to the laboring mother, the PLA has special obstetrical training as a midwife, obstetrical nurse, or laywoman with training in midwifery. We believe that the PLA's knowledge of and experience with birthing, along with her sole focus on the mother's needs, make her a unique and indispensable part of a hospital birth.

The PLA coaches, counsels, supports, and anchors a laboring woman, helping the process move quickly and comfortably. She also acts as an advocate for the mother with the hospital staff, conveying her wishes and freeing her to focus on the labor and imminent birth.

Studies show that woman-supported hospital labors are shorter (by as much as 50 percent) and involve less medical intervention than non-woman-supported hospital labors. In one study, 18 percent of non-woman-supported and 8 percent of woman-supported mothers had cesareans; fewer woman-supported mothers have epidurals, episiotomies, and perineal tears.

PLAs are relatively new players in the birthing game, and few hospitals and insurance companies yet recognize the benefits gained from using professional labor support. For that reason, you may end up paying for a PLA yourself—fees range from $100 to $1200. The average cost is about $300. Negotiate with your insurance carrier if you can, but don't hesitate to take the money out of savings if you have to. PLAs are often instrumental if mothers choose to avoid medical interventions (for example, IV, epidural, and internal fetal monitoring). They are especially valuable in high-risk pregnancies, where the necessary use of such technology makes natural methods of pain control much harder to use. Most important, they aid immeasurably in getting a mother to relax and work with her birthing body.

Be sure to interview PLAs as you would any other professional. Remember that you must be able to trust this woman in order to get the most out of her services. Once you've chosen your PLA, she will schedule a meeting or two during your third trimester to help you work out a realistic birth plan. Most PLAs will next meet you at the hospital once you are in labor, but some will come to your home and help you labor there until it is time to leave for the hospital.

For information on PLAs, contact Doulas of North America (DONA), 13513 North Grove Drive, Alpine, UT 84004 (801-756-7331; fax 801-763-1847; Web site: www.dona.com).

✐

Baby Stools

Q *Someone told me that I can tell if my baby is getting enough to eat by keeping track of his stools. Is this true? How many stools are enough for a newborn?*

A One of the ways to tell if baby is getting enough to eat is to keep track of the frequency and nature of his stools. But first you need to know the normal pattern for newborn stools.

- *First few days.* Baby's stools are black because they are composed primarily of meconium, a black, sticky substance made up of amniotic-fluid debris from his intestines.
- *First week.* Baby's stools change from black to green to brown to yellow.
- *Second week.* Baby's stools take on a more yellowish brown color.
- *First three months.* As baby grows, the number of his daily bowel movements often decreases to an average of one or two a day.

Breastfed Babies

If you are breastfeeding, during the second week your infant should have two to three stools a day that are yellow, seedy, and mustardlike in addition to the yellow-brown stools mentioned above. The yellow stools are a sign that your baby is getting enough of the high-calorie, fatty portion of your milk that helps him grow best.

In part because of breast milk's natural laxative effect, breastfed babies tend to have more frequent stools (two to five per day) than nonbreastfed babies do. These stools are soft and yellow and may have an odor similar to buttermilk. An occasional green stool is not significant as long as your baby is healthy. After the newborn period, the occasional breastfed baby will go one or two days without a bowel movement.

Formula-Fed Babies

The stools of formula-fed babies tend to be less frequent, firmer, darker, and greenish, and usually have an unpleasant odor. You can tell if your choice of formula is agreeing with your baby by observing your infant's stools. If the stools are hard, difficult to pass, and infrequent, your doctor may suggest that you experiment with other formulas that are more intestines friendly.

Other Indicators

The frequency and nature of your infant's stools are two indications of whether or not he is getting enough to eat. If your baby has one or two stools a day but is gaining weight normally and seems content, this may be his normal bowel pattern, while other infants may normally have three to six stools a day. Here are other signs your baby is getting enough to eat.

- She sleeps at least three to four hours at a time.
- She is gaining adequate weight—an average of 1½ pounds during the first month.
- Her skin is not loose or wrinkly, which would occur if she were not putting on enough body fat.

❧

Good Health for Bottlefed Babies

Q *For medical reasons I will not be able to breastfeed my baby. What extra precautions can I take to ensure my baby's health and meet her nutritional needs?*

A Your doctor can help you choose the right formula to meet your baby's nutritional needs. In addition, there are many other things you can do to promote your baby's physical and nutritional health.

- *Eat well during pregnancy.* Nurturing your baby begins in the womb. Take good nutritional care of yourself during your pregnancy to give your unborn baby a healthy start. You'll find useful information about a complete program of nutrition and exercise in *The Pregnancy Book* (Little, Brown, 1997).
- *Stay in touch.* Research shows that touching and interacting with a baby stimulate physical, emotional, and intellectual health. Hold your infant as much as you can during the first year, providing much eye-to-eye and skin-to-skin contact. This physical closeness will enhance your connection with your little one and help your baby get smart from the start.
- *Make feedings special.* Two aspects of the breastfeeding relationship contribute to an infant's sense of well-being: the nutrients in the milk itself; and the increased holding that breastfed babies receive. As well as delivering nutrition, feeding is a social interaction. When bottle-feeding, cuddle your baby as much as you would if you were nursing.
- *Wear your baby in a sling.* In addition to providing physical contact, the motion of being carried will enhance your little one's growth by providing the calming effects of movement.
- *Share sleep.* Sleeping with your baby provides the security of nighttime touch and enhances emotional development. This is especially important for parents who work outside the home. High-touch nighttime parenting will allow you to reconnect with your baby at night and make up for missed touch time during the day.

Above all, respond to your baby's cues in a nurturing way. Ignore any advice to let your baby cry it out. The key word for infant development is "responsiveness."

Years ago at an annual meeting of the American Academy of Pediatrics, Dr. Michael Lewis, Professor of Pediatrics at Rutgers University, reported that after reviewing all the scientific studies on what makes babies smarter and healthier, he found the most important factor to be the caregivers' responsiveness to the baby's cues.

The parenting style you choose is crucial to your infant's development, and attachment parenting (described on pages 45 to 48) is the best way to give your baby the healthiest start possible.

⁊

Baby Formula

Q *I don't plan to breastfeed. How do I pick the best formula for my baby?*

A Human milk is certainly the best nutrition for your baby, but there are medical and lifestyle circumstances in which breastfeeding is not an option. In making formula, manufacturers follow the basic recipe for human milk, which includes proteins, fats, carbohydrates, vitamins, minerals, and water. These ingredients are put into formula in about the same proportions as are in human milk. These nutritional elements are derived either from cow's milk or soybeans. Most formulas are cow's milk–based, which means the basic nutritional building blocks of proteins, fats, and carbohydrates are taken from cow's milk. For infants who are intolerant of or allergic to cow's milk–based formulas, soybeans are an alternative source of adequate nutrition. The standard formulas that you will find on the supermarket shelves (usually varieties of Similac, Enfamil, Carnation, and the newer store brands) are similar in nutritional content, and all these formulas have to meet rigid government standards for adequate infant nutrition.

Consult your doctor before selecting the formula for your baby. Until recently parents relied only on their baby's doctor to choose the right formula. It was considered unethical for formula companies to advertise directly to consumers. Recently this code of nutritional ethics has been violated by some formula companies advertising directly to parents. The American Academy of Pediatrics has wisely condemned this practice. As you would do with any medicine that goes into your baby, consult your baby's doctor in choosing a formula.

While formula companies are constantly updating the nutritional quality of infant formulas, as a parent who wants to give her infant the best nutritional start, you should be aware of the fact that infant formulas made in America lack an essential brain-building fat called DHA. While human milk is rich in DHA, formulas made in America do not have DHA, unlike formulas manufactured in nearly all other developed countries. Many researchers attribute the intellectual advantages of breastfeeding to the presence of DHA. In light of this new research on the importance of DHA as a vital brain-building fat, some American formula companies are currently considering adding this vital fat. For an update on DHA-enriched formulas made in America, consult our Web site DHAdoc.com.

If you choose to feed your newborn formula, be sure to observe the following safe formula-feeding procedures:

- Use formula before the expiration date on the label.
- Use refrigerated, opened, ready-to-feed, and prepared formula within forty-eight hours.
- Don't leave bottles of formula out of the refrigerator for more than two hours.
- Throw away the formula left in the bottle after a feeding, since germs from baby's saliva will multiply in the warm formula.
- Refrigerate any formula saved from one day to the next.
- It's best not to heat formula in a microwave. Because of uneven heating, hot spots develop. If you do use the microwave, shake the bottle well before testing the temperature on your wrist; or place the bottle inside a mug filled with microwave-heated water and swirl the bottle often to even the heat. For more on concerns about microwaving breast milk, see page 81.
- Avoid bottle propping, and don't let a baby fall asleep holding his bottle. He could choke or aspirate the formula into his lungs. Falling asleep with a bottle allows the sugary formula to pool in the mouth, in contact with teeth, causing tooth decay. Also, when a baby feeds from a bottle in the lying-down position, formula may travel from the back of the baby's throat up through the eustachian tube into the middle ear, causing ear infections.

Remember that bottlefeeding, like breastfeeding, is a social interaction, in addition to a method of delivering nutrition. There should always be a person at both ends of the bottle, and babies should go to sleep attached to a person, not a bottle.

☙

From Womb-Mate to Roommate

Q *I'm so worried that I won't feel that bond with my baby that everyone talks about. How do I go about making that connection with my baby after she's born?*

A　"Bonding"—the term for the close emotional tie that develops between parents and baby at birth—was the buzzword of the eighties. Dr. Marshall H. Klaus and Dr. John H. Kennell explored the concept in their classic book entitled *Bonding: The Beginnings of Parent-Infant Attachment.* These researchers speculated that for humans, just as for other types of animals, there is a "sensitive period" right after birth when mothers and newborns are uniquely programmed to be in contact with each other and do good things to each other. By comparing mother-infant pairs who bonded immediately after birth with those who didn't, they concluded that the early-contact mother-infant pairs later developed a closer attachment.

Bonding is not a now-or-never phenomenon. Bonding during this biologically sensitive period does give the parent-infant relationship a head start. But immediate bonding after birth is not like instant glue that cements a parent-child relationship forever. The overselling of bonding has caused needless guilt for mothers who, because of a medical complication, were temporarily separated from their babies after birth. Epidemics of bonding blues have occurred in mothers who had cesarean births or whose premature babies stayed for a time in intensive care units.

Here are some easy tips to encourage better bonding with baby:

- *Delay routine procedures.* Oftentimes the attending nurse does routine procedures, gives the vitamin K shot, and instills eye ointment in baby's eyes immediately after birth and then presents baby to mother for bonding. Ask the nurse to delay these procedures for an hour or so, until your new baby has enjoyed the initial bonding period. The eye ointment temporarily blurs baby's vision or causes her eyes to stay closed. She needs a clear first impression of you, and you need to see those eyes.
- *Stay connected.* Ask your birth attendant and nurses to put your baby on your abdomen and chest immediately after birth or after cutting the cord and suctioning your baby, unless a medical complication requires temporary separation.
- *Let your baby breastfeed right after birth.* Most babies are content simply to lick the nipple; others have a strong desire to suck at the breast immediately after birth. This nipple stimulation releases the hormone oxytocin, which increases the contractions of your uterus and lessens postpartum bleeding. Early sucking also stimulates the release of prolactin, the hormone that helps your mothering abilities click in right from the start.
- *Room-in with your baby.* Of course bonding does not end at the delivery bed—it is just the beginning! Making visual, tactile, olfactory, auditory, and sucking connection with your baby right after the birth may make you feel you don't want to release this little person that you have labored so hard to bring into the world—and

you don't have to. Your womb-mate can now become your roommate. We advise healthy mothers and healthy babies to remain together throughout their hospital stay.

Some babies make a stable transition from womb to world without any complications; others need a few hours in the nursery for extra warmth, oxygen, suctioning, and other special attention until their vital systems stabilize. Then they can return to the nursery of mother's arms.

- *Touch your baby.* Besides providing stimulation for your baby from the skin-to-skin contact of tummy-to-tummy and cheek-to-breast, gently stroke your baby, caressing his whole body. We have noticed that mothers and fathers often caress their babies differently. A new mother usually strokes her baby's entire body with a gentle caress of her fingertips; the new father often places an entire hand on his baby's head, as if symbolizing his commitment to protect the life he has fathered. Besides being enjoyable, stroking the skin is medically beneficial to the newborn. The skin, the largest organ in the human body, is very rich with nerve endings. At the time when baby is making the transition to air breathing and the initial breathing patterns are very irregular, stroking stimulates the newborn to breathe more rhythmically— the therapeutic value of a parent's touch.

- *Gaze at your newborn.* Your newborn can see you best with an eye-to-eye distance of 8 to 10 inches (20 to 25 centimeters)—amazingly, about the usual nipple-to-eye distance during breastfeeding. Place your baby in the face-to-face position, adjusting your head and your baby's head in the same position so that your eyes meet. Enjoy this visual connection during the brief period of quiet alertness after birth, before baby falls into a deep sleep. Staring into your baby's eyes may trigger a rush of beautiful mothering feelings.

- *Talk to your newborn.* During the first hours and days after birth, a natural baby-talk dialogue will develop between mother and infant. Voice-analysis studies have shown a unique rhythm and comforting cadence to mother's voice.

Feelings after birth are as individual as feelings after lovemaking. Many mothers show the immediate glow of motherhood and the "birth high" excitement of a race finished and won. It's love at first sight, and they can't wait to get their hands on their baby and begin mothering within a millisecond after birth. Others are relieved that the mammoth task of birth is over, that baby is normal. Now they are more interested in sleeping and recovering than bonding and mothering. As one mother said, following a lengthy and arduous labor, "Let me sleep for a few hours, take a shower, comb my hair, and then I'll start mothering." If these are your feelings, enjoy your rest—you've earned it. There is no need to succumb to the pressure to bond when neither your body nor your mind is willing or able. In this case, Father bonds while Mother rests.

The important thing is that someone is bonding during this sensitive period of one to two hours of quiet alertness after birth. One of the saddest sights we see is a newly born baby parked all alone in the nursery, busily bonding (with wide-open, hungry eyes) with the plastic sides of her bassinet. Give your baby a significant presence—mother, father, or even grandma in a pinch.

$\mathscr{L\!\!\!\!\!\!\!\!\!\!\!\!\!\!\!\!D}$

Bonding with Your Preemie

Q *I just had a premature baby, and because she's still in an incubator, I'm worried that my partner and I are missing out on valuable bonding time. What can we do to start the process now?*

A   It's easy for parents of a premature infant to feel displaced by the medical team, but remember, you are vital team members. A premature baby's response to her mother's and father's touch is something medical science can never duplicate—and it can speed your baby's growth. While your baby is still in the incubator, gently stroke her. Studies have shown that this so-called healing touch helps preemies grow better.

You can also practice a therapy called "kangaroo care," which simulates the nurturing environment of the womb. As soon as your baby outgrows her need for oxygen, wear her around the nursery in a sling as much as you can. Or rock with her snuggled against your chest. Skin-to-skin contact is extremely beneficial, so open your blouse and snuggle baby against you. Be sure to wrap a blanket around her.

Research by Dr. Gene Anderson, at Case Western Reserve University in Cleveland, Ohio, reveals kangaroo care may help a baby gain weight faster, have fewer stop-breathing episodes, and experience a shorter hospital stay. Babies who get kangaroo care also cry less—an important benefit, because excessive crying wastes precious oxygen and energy and can keep a premature baby from growing optimally. The rhythm of walking as you wear your baby in a sling will help her breathe more regularly, even more so than rocking her in a chair. After all, she became accustomed to exactly this kind of movement when she was inside you. If you are planning on nursing, the closeness to your breast will stimulate your baby to do so. (Until your baby is ready to breastfeed, you can pump your breast milk to give to your baby. For more information on pumping milk, contact La Leche League, a nationwide breastfeeding support group; see Resources for Childcare Products and Information, page 129).

As for bonding, keep in mind that it's not like glue that instantly cements the mother-infant relationship. Rather, it's a gradual, ongoing process that begins soon after birth and continues throughout life. If you wear your daughter in a sling, nurse her, and give her lots of skin-to-skin contact both while she's in the hospital and after she goes home, you'll be off to a great start with the bonding process.

✍

Baby's First Outing

Q *We've been cooped up in the house for seven days now since coming home from the hospital. How do I know when it is safe to take my baby out for the first time?*

A The main factors that influence how soon after birth baby can go outside are maturity and weight of baby and the weather. Premature and low-birth-weight babies, because they are not born with an excess of insulating body fat, are more sensitive to temperature changes, so it is wise to keep these babies in a consistent temperature of around 68° F to 70° F for the first month.

Going from a heated house to a heated car to another heated house right after birth is safe for a term baby who weighs more than 7 pounds. Also, if the temperature outside is similar to that inside, then certainly your newborn can go outside right away. If your baby is premature, small for date, or under 7 pounds, it would be wise to keep baby's head covered when you're outside in cold weather. The head is one of the main avenues of heat loss for newborns, so it is wise to keep all newborns' heads covered in cold weather for at least the first month.

For mother's and baby's sakes, avoid crowded places for at least the first month. Passersby love to stop and peer at a tiny baby. To avoid unnecessary exposure to germs, shun crowded places (for example, supermarkets, church nurseries, and shopping malls) and handling by people with colds. You need the downtime and rest, and your baby does not need the exposure to germs.

The bottom line? Use common sense. A bit of fresh air is good for newborns and their mommies. As soon as you are up to taking a walk after birth, dress your newborn appropriately, place him securely in a sling, and enjoy a stroll outside—weather permitting.

✐

When It's Time to Call the Doctor

Q *What are the signs that my baby is sick and needs a doctor? I'm afraid that with all of the little quirks newborns have I might miss something important.*

A Get used to how your baby normally acts when well: the sparkle in her eyes, the pink skin color, her happy disposition, and her eating and sleeping patterns. All of these change when babies are sick. The younger the baby, the more subtle the signs, especially in newborns.

Also, get acquainted with your baby's "feel." Notice how her muscle tone is generally firm, and the muscles in her arms and limbs are somewhat tight and spring back easily when you flex them. Newborns' skin is generally pink. Healthy newborns tend to be active and have frequent periods of quiet alertness when they seem attentive to their caregivers.

Some signs of newborn illness that merit medical attention include:

- Increasing drowsiness, paleness, and lethargy and a slower-than-usual response to you.
- Any fever above 101° F (taken rectally) that persists for more than four hours, even after you've dressed baby in lighter clothing.
- A progressive lack of interest in feeding, fewer wet diapers, and dry, wrinkly skin. These are all signs baby is becoming dehydrated.

- Your "mother's intuition" sounding an alarm that your baby just doesn't look, act, and feel right, and after an hour or two of observation you still have this feeling.

Since a newborn's immune system is less mature than that of an older child, the signs of illness are more subtle. This results in illnesses progressing from nonserious to serious more rapidly. In any situation, it is wise to seek medical attention if your newborn appears sick.

✑

Talking Baby Talk

Q *My baby's only a couple of weeks old. Is it too early to think about how her verbal skills are developing? Should I avoid talking baby talk? It seems like normal speech would be better for introducing verbal communication to an infant. I mean, we don't want kids who speak "coochie-coo," right?*

A Have fun with your baby, and one of the wonderful ways for you to enjoy one another is to talk with her. Don't be self-conscious; talk to your baby any way you enjoy. Mothers are natural baby talkers, using a language we call "motherese." They raise the pitch, slow the rate, E-X-A-G-G-E-R-A-T-E the syllables, and instinctively draw out their vowels—"Goooood baaaby."

You may not realize it now, but you are naturally teaching your baby language. Video analysis of the fine art of mother-baby communication shows that mother talks as if she imagines baby talks back. She naturally shortens her messages and elongates her pauses to the exact length of time that coincides with the length of the imagined response from the baby. This is especially true when she is talking to baby in the form of a question.

You might consider this your baby's earliest speech lesson, as you are shaping your baby's ability to listen. Your baby stores these early experiences away and later recalls them when beginning to speak.

When talking to your baby, keep it simple. Use short two- or three-word sentences and one- or two-syllable words with lots of drawn-out, exaggerated vowels ("Preeetty baaaby"). As when composing a telegram, avoid cluttering your dialogue with "the" and "a." Drop the pronouns "I" and "me." They have no meaning to a baby. Refer to yourselves as "Mommy" and "Daddy."

As your baby grows, keep your speech lively. As you say, "Wave bye-bye cat," wave your hands in a bye-bye gesture at the cat. Baby is more likely to recall words that are associated with animated gestures. Give your speech some spark with some inflections at the end of the sentence, and exaggerate important words.

Give a running commentary of your daily maintenance tasks, such as diaper changing, bathing, and dressing, much like a sportscaster describing a game: "Now Daddy takes off the diaper . . . now we put on a new one . . ." Sure, it's normal to feel a bit foolish initially, but you are not talking to a stone wall! There is a little person with big ears processing every word she hears and storing it on an endless memory record.

☞

7 Ways to Relax a Fussy Baby

Q *I had a baby two weeks ago, and the house hasn't been quiet since. What are the best ways for calming a crying baby?*

A Babies fuss and parents comfort. That's a realistic fact of new family life. It helps to understand what calms a baby and why. Most calming techniques involve at least one of these four interactions:

- rhythmic motion
- soothing sounds
- visual delights and distractions
- close physical contact and touching

Calming techniques (except visual ones) are like re-creating the womb that baby has been used to for nine months. Here are seven baby-calming techniques that worked with our own fussy babies and that we have learned from experienced baby-calmers in our pediatric practice. Remember, your baby has individual needs. Try these techniques as a starting point and improvise. After a few months, you and your baby will have a large repertoire of fuss-busters that work.

1. Wear your baby in a sling. A baby carrier will be your most useful fuss-preventing tool. Infant-development researchers who study baby-care practices in America and other cultures report unanimously that *infants who are car-*

ried more cry less. In fact, research has shown that babies who are carried at least three hours a day cry 40 percent less than infants who aren't carried as much. Over the years in pediatric practice, I have listened to and watched veteran baby-calmers and heard this recurrent theme: "As long as I have my baby in my arms or on my body, she's content." This observation led us to coin the term "baby-wearing." Babywearing means more than just picking up baby and putting him in a carrier when he fusses. It means carrying baby many hours a day *before* he needs to fuss. This means the carrier you choose must be easy to use and versatile. We have found the sling-type carrier to be the most conducive to babywearing. The sling becomes part of your apparel, and you can easily wear your baby in the sling several hours a day. Mothers who do this tell us their babies seem to forget to fuss.

2. Dance with your baby. It's only natural that movement calms fussy babies. Their whole uterine existence was definitely one moving experience! Babies crave movement after birth because to them it is the norm. Being still disconcerts babies. They don't understand it, and it frightens them. Movement relaxes them.

3. Swing your baby. Walk past any playground or peer into any nursery, and you'll see happy babies swinging contentedly. The regular swinging motion calms babies. To meet the high demands of fussy babies and frantic parents, infant-product manufacturers have introduced a variety of baby swings to the ever-growing market of baby-soothing devices. None of these synthetic substitutes works as well as the encircling arms, soft breasts, or warm body of a parent, all of which remind baby of the womb, but let's face it, substitute arms are sometimes necessary to save a parent's sanity or at least allow mother to take a shower. Swings are particularly useful during "happy hour," that stretch of time in the late afternoon to early evening when you're busy preparing or having dinner and babies are notoriously difficult. Be sure to buy a swing approved by the Juvenile Products Manufacturers Association (JPMA). Mechanical swings are one of the most commonly recalled infant products. Used swings or swings bought at second-hand stores may not contain proper safety harnesses.

4. Try freeway fathering (or mothering). If you've tried several of the home-based tricks to settle baby and none has worked, take a ride. Place baby in a car seat and drive for at least twenty minutes, nonstop if you can. Then return home and carry the whole package (sleeping baby in the car seat) into your home. I used freeway fathering at times to give Martha a much-needed baby break. Sometimes Martha and I would take a drive together for some couple-communication time as our moving baby drifted off to sleep. Sometimes I would bring a pillow along, and after our baby fell asleep in the backseat, I would return to our driveway, park, and stretch out on the front seat for a bit of recharging before daily life put more demands on me.

5. Take a carriage stroll. For many modern mothers, wearing babies in carriers has replaced pushing them in carriages. Certainly babies would give two thumbs up to this improved mode of travel. However, while most babies settle better when worn than when wheeled, some high-need babies like a change of scenery and sometimes settle better in a carriage or stroller. Some infants shun the flimsy, hard, rough-riding collapsible strollers and prefer the old-fashioned, cushy, bouncy (and expensive!) prams. That's typical of high-need children.

6. Roll your baby. Kneel on the floor and drape baby tummy-down over a beach ball. Hold baby with one hand and slightly roll the ball from side to side.

7. Walk with your baby. One of the easiest baby- and

parent-calmers is a simple walk. When our babies were fussy and obviously needed a change of scenery, I borrowed a motto from Knute Rockne, the famous Notre Dame football coach: "When the going gets tough, the tough get going." Martha or I would nestle our baby in a sling and take a long walk, frequently varying the route and the attractions. We would walk past moving cars, moving people, trees, parks, children playing, up and down hills, along curving paths, and oftentimes along the beach. Sometimes Martha and I began the day with a baby walk, which seemed to start the day off better for both of us. Other times, when our babies were going through the stage when they fussed a lot around dinnertime, we would take a walk around 5:00 P.M. This mellowed them out enough that they would reward us by forgetting to fuss that evening. Besides calming fussy babies, long, pleasant walks are good exercise for parents.

Keeping Baby Warm

Q *I'm not sure how warm I need to keep my newborn. What's the right temperature for a nursery? And how should I dress her?*

A Besides a consistent temperature of around 68° to 70° F, the humidity level in the bedroom is important, too. The best humidity level is around 60 to 70 percent. Less humidity may dry out a baby's breathing passages, making her nose stuffy and thickening the mucus in the airways. High humidity, on the other hand, favors the growth of respiratory allergens and may peel off the paint or wallpaper. Central heating is not friendly to tiny breathing passages, because the air is either too dry or full of allergens.

Here's a healthier alternative: Turn the central heating down during the night and turn on a warm-mist vaporizer in baby's bedroom. Because steam kills bacteria, it is healthier than cool mist. This inexpensive steam producer (available at pharmacies and infant-product stores for around $10) provides two benefits: It increases the humidity in the room, and it warms the room.

From high school physics you know that when steam condenses, it releases heat. That's how a vaporizer warms the room. (**Safety tip:** As baby reaches the grabbing stage, keep hot-mist vaporizers out of baby's reach.)

Consider three factors when dressing your baby for sleep: comfort, warmth, and safety. What style and fabric are most comfortable to your baby is a matter of observation. It won't take you long to figure out whether your baby sleeps better in footed sleepers or loose, tie-at-the-bottom sacques. Learning how to dress your baby appropriately is really only a matter of common sense and getting a feel for your individual baby. Also, an appropriately clothed baby is more likely to reward you with a less disturbed night's sleep. Overheated infants tend to be more restless.

As a general guide, dress and cover your infant in as much or as little clothing and blankets as you would put on yourself. Then feel your baby's head or the back of her neck. If these areas feel too hot or if baby is sweating, remove one layer. If baby feels cold, add a layer. In general, it's safer to adjust your baby's sleeping temperature by changing clothes than by piling on more blankets. Baby's hands and feet are not accurate indicators of body temperature since, in most babies, these parts are usually cooler than the rest of the body.

Consider these tips and precautions:

- *Sleepers with feet are the most practical.* Even if baby kicks off his blankets, you can be sure he has one layer of warmth. A minor drawback to sleepers is that it's harder to get a good fit in a one-piece garment. Still, they don't need to fit perfectly. Buy them loose since they are quickly outgrown.
- *Try cotton sleepwear.* Most of our babies seemed more comfortable (and had fewer irritating rashes) in cotton sleepwear, which absorbs moisture and "breathes," or allows air to circulate freely. Since cotton sleepwear allows for the release of body heat, it lessens the chance of baby becoming overheated. Flame-retardant cotton sleepwear is now available, but it may be more difficult to find than polyester.
- *Dress your baby in the proper size.* Make sure that sleepwear is loose enough to allow her to move freely but snug enough to stay on the right body parts.

✍

Boosting a Newborn's IQ

Q *My two-week-old seems so tiny and sleepy. Should I be doing anything to keep her stimulated when she's awake? Is there anything I can do to make her smarter?*

A "Smart-from-the-start parenting" means basically helping the infant's developing brain make the right connections. New insights into how a baby's brain grows show that parents have a profound effect on their child's ability to learn.

The brain grows more during infancy than at any other time, doubling its volume and reaching approximately 60 percent of its adult size by one year. As the brain grows, nerve cells called neurons proliferate, resembling miles of tangled electrical wires. The infant is born with much of this wiring unconnected. During the first year, these neurons grow larger, learn to work better, and connect with each other to make circuits that enable baby to think and do more things.

Here's how these circuits work. The tips of each neuron resemble fingerlike feelers ready to make connections with other nerves. As the brain develops, two important improvements are made on the beginning nervous system: The number of connections between neurons increases, and each neuron acquires a coating called myelin, which helps the messages move faster and insulates the nerve, preventing short circuits. The new and exciting field of neurobiology tells us that the more connections the nerve cells make, the smarter the child's brain is.

Inhaling or ingesting substances called neurotoxins, such as cigarette smoke, excessive amounts of alcohol, and certain drugs, has been shown to harm brain development and increase a child's risk of developing learning and behavior problems later. To balance out the don'ts of drugs, alcohol, and nicotine during pregnancy, there are some vital dos that affect the developing fetal brain in a healthy way. Here are some simple ways you can help your baby become smarter:

- *Smart nutritional start.* Breast milk gives baby a head start. At least seven scientific studies show that breastfed babies are smarter than bottlefed, and the more frequently and longer infants are breastfed, the greater their intellectual advantage. The increased cognitive development that breastfed babies enjoy is due not only to the increase in nurturing and touch they receive (which bottlefeeding mothers can do, too!), but also to the brain-building fats (especially DHA) in breast milk, which provide the components for building myelin, the insulating sheath around nerve fibers that helps messages travel faster. Researchers agree that it's the "smart fats" in breast milk that contribute to this intellectual advantage.

- *Smart carrying.* Carried babies show an increase in awake time called quiet alertness. This is the behavioral state in which an infant is most content and best able to interact with the environment. Carried babies receive more attentive parenting and more interaction with their environment, which encourages more brain cell connections. (See page 6.)

- *Smart talk.* How you speak to your baby has a profound effect on her brain development. Here's where parents, especially mothers, really shine. Moms are naturals when it comes to communicating with infants, instinctively adopting the upbeat tones and facial gestures of motherese. In fact, you probably already naturally raise your pitch, s-l-o-w your rate of speaking, and E-X-A-G-G-E-R-A-T-E your vowels and syllables when addressing your baby ("Preeetty baaaby!"). Notice that when you talk to your baby, you put your entire face into the act by widening your mouth and eyes while talking. You naturally slow down and speed up according to baby's attention. How a mother talks to her baby is more important than what she actually says.

• *Smart responses.* Responding to a baby's cues builds brain connections. It's not only how you talk to your infant but also how you listen that helps to build a brainy baby. Many studies show that the most powerful enhancer of brain development is the quality of parent-infant attachment and the response of the caregiving environment to the cues of the infant. A high-touch, high-response style of parenting promotes baby brain development by feeding the brain the right kind of information at a time in the child's life when the brain needs the most nourishment. If you are beginning to feel important in helping build your baby's brain, you are! Simply stated, the volumes of new research conclude that parents are crucial in making a baby smarter. Not so long ago parents were bombarded with the wrong message that what they bought for baby was more important for intellectual stimulation than what they did with baby. A parental overreaction to consumer overmarketing resulted in nurseries being filled with so many black-and-white toys and mobiles that they looked like bedrooms for baby zebras. Infant-stimulation classes mushroomed and brain-stimulation toys were promoted to parents seeking a head start to Harvard for their children.

There is no evidence that fancy toys and expensive classes make brighter babies. When researchers compared the influence of toys and programs on infant development with responsive parenting, mothers still came out on top. In the keynote address at the 1986 annual meeting of the American Academy of Pediatrics, infant-development specialist Dr. Michael Lewis reviewed the studies of factors that build brighter babies. His presentation was in response to the overselling of the "superbaby" phenomenon, which emphasized the use of programs and kits that coaxed parents into the role of teachers rather than playful companions and sensitive nurturers. Lewis concluded that the single most important influence on a child's intellectual development is the responsiveness of the caregivers to the cues of the child. Cues build connections. So it isn't the stuff you buy or the cards you flash that give baby a smart start. Rather, it's healthy, responsive parent-child relationships.

♋

A Newborn's Appearance

Q *My husband and I were touring a maternity ward recently and noticed that none of the newborn babies looked anything like baby pictures you see in magazines. What's the deal?*

A You're right! None of the newly born babies in the nursery look like those pictured in magazines. That's because those in the magazines are older newborns, who are neatly dressed and groomed. Newly born babies—and their mothers—look like they have been through a lot of long hard work, which is called labor. Some mothers have described their newly born babies as looking like a prizefighter—after the fight.

When you examine your baby in the first hour after birth, you will find him beautiful. Here is the appearance you can expect. Baby's puffy face and eyelids are a result of extra fluid accumulated beneath the skin. He will show some signs of having had to squeeze a bit to enter the world. His face has areas of bluish purple, dotted with freckled spots from tiny broken blood vessels. Several other characteristics of the face and head give further evidence of baby's tight squeeze through the birth canal: a flattened nose, ears pressed against the head, and a slight bruising of the skin.

The watermelon shape of your baby's head is the result of a process called molding, which helps your baby's head fit through the pelvic bones during delivery and protects the underlying brain. The top of your baby's skull is made up of five bones that are joined together by tough membranes. As your baby's head moves through the birth canal, these bones move and allow the head to elongate to conform more easily to the shape of the birth canal. Because of the molding, your baby's head is larger and longer in the back, and his forehead appears relatively flat. The skull bones may overlap a bit and you may feel ridges on the bones, especially on the top and sides of baby's head. This normal molding gives many newborns a conehead appearance. Within twenty-four hours after birth, your baby's head assumes a smoother, rounder shape. Molding is more noticeable after longer labors and in babies with larger heads.

You'll also notice that your newborn's scalp is swollen, and occasionally tiny blood vessels beneath the scalp may break during delivery, allowing blood to accumulate and form a sort of goose egg on baby's scalp. This is called a cephalohematoma (see page 96). The bump may take several months to disappear and may sometimes feel very hard as the underlying blood calcifies.

A fine, silky baby hair, matted with amniotic fluid and specks of blood, covers your baby's head right after birth. You will also notice patches of fine, fuzzy hair called lanugo on baby's earlobes, cheeks, shoulders, and upper back.

Your newborn's beautiful skin is covered with a white, cheesy, slippery material called vernix, which protects it from the amniotic fluid and acts like a lubricant during vaginal delivery. Naturally, all this stuff is wiped off before those baby pictures you see in the magazine. You'll be amazed at how quickly the head, face, and skin change in your newly born baby, and within a week your beauty will look similar to the babies in magazines.

✑

Newborn Skin

Q *I'm concerned about some strange markings on my baby's face. What are the common newborn skin conditions?*

A Infants seldom have picture-perfect skin in the first few months. One of the earliest skin conditions you will notice is newborn acne, facial pimples that erupt because of hormonal changes. Like teenage acne, the red, pimply, oily rash covers much of baby's face, and the previously soft, smooth cheeks feel sandpaper rough. Newborn acne usually peaks around the third week and clears within a month or six weeks, so hold off on the precious baby pictures until after the acne has cleared.

Another common baby rash is seborrheic dermatitis. This skin condition looks like baby acne, but it occurs in larger patches and is more yellowish and crusty. It is caused by an overproduction of an oily substance called sebum in the oil glands of the skin. This rash is most noticeable on the cheeks, behind the ears, and on the scalp. Red, raised, or rough rashes can also be caused by an allergy to baby's formula or to an allergen in the milk of a breastfeeding mother, such as a dairy product.

Avoid the tendency to overwash newborn rashy skin, as it may worsen. Extensive cleansing, especially with strong soap, will only dry out an infant's sensitive skin. Wash these rashy areas as you normally would with water—only once or twice a week—or perhaps use a mild soap—sparingly—and gently pat dry.

Also in the early months normal spots and specks develop on baby's otherwise beautiful skin. The most common are dubbed "stork bites." These are reddish pink marks that are most common on the eyelids, the nape of the neck, and the middle of the forehead. These reddish marks often "light up" when baby cries. These curious blotches are caused by blood vessels showing through the newborn's thin skin. As your baby's skin thickens, the marks fade, usually by baby's first birthday. Some of these pink blotches may remain on the nape of the neck, but they are obscured by hair.

Also expect a reddish pimply rash called prickly heat. This appears in moist areas of the skin, especially between the neck folds, behind the ears, in the groin, and in areas where clothing fits tightly. To take the heat and the prickles out of the rash, dress your baby in lightweight, loose-fitting cotton clothing and gently wash the skin with plain cool water or a solution of baking soda (1 teaspoon to 8 ounces of water). Dab the rashy areas and blot dry. Be careful not to scrub or harshly rub the sensitive skin of young infants. A safe and effective emollient and lubricant for an infant's dry, sensitive, rashy skin is Soothe and Heal with Lansinoh.

Also common, especially in infants of African, Asian, Latino, and East Indian descent, are black-and-blue marks on baby's lower back and buttocks. These spots often fade with time, but many never completely disappear.

ॐ

The Facts About Attachment Parenting

Q *You talk frequently about attachment parenting. Exactly what does this term mean, and how does it benefit baby and parents?*

A Attachment parenting is a style of caring for your infant that brings out what we call the "baby B's"—the best in baby and parents. There are six principal concepts that make up attachment parenting:

1. Birth bonding. The way babies and parents get started helps the early attachment unfold. The days and weeks after birth are a sensitive period when mother and baby are uniquely primed to want to be close to each other. A close attachment after birth and beyond allows the natural, biological attachment-promoting behaviors of the infant and the intuitive, biological caregiving qualities of the mother to come together. Both members of this biological pair get off to the right start at a time when the infant is most needy and the mother is most ready to nurture.

2. Breastfeeding. Breastfeeding is an exercise in baby reading, meaning, it helps you read your baby's cues or body language, which is the first step in getting to know your baby. Breastfeeding promotes the right chemistry between the mother and baby by stimulating your body to produce prolactin and oxytocin, hormones that give your mothering a boost.

3. Babywearing. A baby learns a lot in the arms of a busy caregiver. Carried babies fuss less and spend more time in a state of quiet alertness, the behavior state most conducive to learning and interaction. Babywearing improves the sensitivity of the parents, too. Because your baby is so close to you, you get to know her better. Closeness promotes familiarity.

4. Bedding close to baby. While it's crucial that all family members get the best night's sleep possible, co-sleeping adds a nighttime touch that helps busy daytime parents reconnect with their infant at night. Sleeping within close touching and nursing distance minimizes nighttime separation anxiety and helps baby learn that sleep is a pleasant state to enter and a fearless state in which to remain.

5. Belief in the meaning of your baby's cry. Babies cry to communicate, not to manipulate. Responding sensitively to your baby's cries builds a trust that goes both ways: Babies learn to trust that their caregivers will be responsive to their needs, and parents gradually learn to trust their ability to meet these needs. This raises the parent-child communication level a notch.

6. Being wary of baby trainers. Attachment parenting teaches you how to be discerning of advice, especially those rigid and extreme parenting styles that teach you to watch a clock or a schedule instead of your baby. This "convenience parenting" may be a short-term gain, but it's a long-term loss and not a wise investment. These more restrained styles of parenting create a distance between you and your baby and keep you from becoming an expert in *your* child.

Attachment Parenting Is a Starter Style

These six baby B's help parents and baby get off to the right start. Use them as starter tips to work out your own parenting style—one that fits the individual needs of your child and your family. If there are medical or family circumstances that keep you from practicing all of the baby B's, remember that attachment parenting means opening your mind and heart to the individual needs of your baby, and eventually you will develop the wisdom to make on-the-spot decisions about what works best for both of you. Do the best you can with the resources you have—that's all your child will ever expect of you.

Attachment Parenting Is an Approach

Rather than a strict set of rules, attachment parenting is a style of parenting, and one that many people instinctively lean toward. But parenting is too individual and your baby is too complex for there to be only one way. The important point is that you get connected to your baby, and the baby B's of attachment parenting help you do that. Once connected, stick with what is working and modify what is not. You will ultimately develop your own parenting style that helps you and baby find a way to get to know each other.

Attachment Parenting Is
Responsive Parenting

By becoming sensitive to the cues of your infant, you learn to read your baby's level of need. When baby learns that

his needs will be met and his language listened to, he
learns to trust his ability to give cues. As a result, baby
becomes a better cue giver, parents become better cue
readers, and the whole parent-child communication net-
work becomes easier.

⚘

Gas Bubbles vs. Smiley Face

Q *My baby's only three weeks old, but it really looks
like he's smiling at me. This couldn't be just gas, could it?*

A Adults don't smile because of gas, and neither do
babies. So let's deflate the gas bubble! The smiles occurring in the first few weeks are a beautiful reflection of
your baby's inner feelings of rightness. Some are sleep
grins. Some are only a happy twitch at the corner of their
mouth. Relief smiles occur after being rescued from a
colicky period, after a satisfying feeding, or after being
picked up and rocked. You are most likely to catch a
smile when you play face-to-face games. Baby's early
smiles convey "I feel good inside," and that should leave
you feeling good inside, too. These early fleeting grins
are glimpses of the whole happy-face smiles that will
come next month.

Whereas the smiles of the first month are reflex
smiles, automatic reactions to an inner feeling of rightness and limited to the muscles of the mouth, the smiles
your baby gives you in the second month are real social

smiles in response to your smile and facial gestures.
Baby's whole face lights up. Her eyes are wide open and,
if she is really into it, crinkled up at the corners. Dimples
appear in baby's chubby cheeks as she flashes her tooth-
less grins. Typically, smiles progress from fleeting grins
in the first month to facial smiles in the second month to
smiles and total body wiggles during smile games at three
to four months.

Remember, smiling is a two-way communication game
between the smiler and the smilee. When you spot your
baby's smiles, smile back. Jazz up your smile to intensify
baby's smile. These first smiles reward you so much and
are so beautiful that you'll momentarily forget the sleep
you are losing and your social and professional life that is
now on hold.

✑

Breast vs. Bottle

Q *Does breast milk really make such a difference? I
want to do what's best for my baby, but I'm just not comfortable with all the work and inconvenience that accom-
panies nursing. I was bottlefed, and I turned out fine.*

A Yes, breast milk does make a difference. One of the
greatest gifts you can give your baby is your milk. The
American Academy of Pediatrics recommends that mothers breastfeed for at least one year. If there are medical or
lifestyle reasons that you can't breastfeed for that long,

breastfeed your baby for as long as you can. Giving your baby your milk for even a few weeks or a few months gives your infant the best nutritional start.

Breastfeeding Benefits Baby

Breastfeeding is good for every part of baby's body, from top to bottom. Here is a list of the benefits of breastfeeding that are validated by scientific research:

- *Brain.* Breastfed children have higher IQs. The special types of omega-3 fats in human milk enhance the growth of nerve tissue.
- *Eyes.* Visual acuity is higher in babies fed human milk.
- *Ears.* Breastfed babies get fewer ear infections.
- *Mouth.* There is less need for orthodontic work in children who were breastfed for more than a year. Sucking at the breast leads to improved muscle development of the face. Subtle changes in the taste of human milk prepare babies to accept a variety of solid foods.
- *Throat.* Children who were breastfed are less likely to require tonsillectomies. Breastfeeding also offers protection against the effects of hypothyroidism.
- *Respiratory system.* Breastfed babies have fewer and less severe upper-respiratory infections, less wheezing, less pneumonia, and less influenza.
- *Heart and circulatory system.* Breastfed children may have lower cholesterol levels as adults. Heart rates are lower in breastfed infants.
- *Digestive system.* Babies who are breastfeeding have less diarrhea and fewer gastrointestinal infections. Six months or more of exclusive breastfeeding reduces baby's risk of later developing Crohn's disease and

ulcerative colitis. Breastfeeding can continue during a
gastrointestinal illness.
- *Immune system.* Breastfed babies respond better to vac-
  cinations. Human milk helps to mature baby's immune
  system. Breastfeeding decreases the risk of childhood
  cancers and juvenile diabetes.
- *Kidneys.* With less salt and less protein than formula,
  human milk is easier on a baby's kidneys.
- *Appendix.* Children who were breastfed are unlikely to
  develop acute appendicitis.
- *Urinary tract.* Breastfed infants have fewer urinary tract
  infections.
- *Joints and muscles.* Juvenile rheumatoid arthritis is less
  common in children who were breastfed.
- *Skin.* There is less incidence of allergic eczema among
  breastfed infants.
- *Growth.* Breastfed babies are leaner at one year of age
  and less likely to be obese later in life.
- *Diapers.* Breastfed babies are less constipated, and their
  stools are less offensive in odor.

Breastfeeding Benefits Mothers, Too!

Breastfeeding mothers enjoy a reduced risk of breast, uterine, and ovarian cancer, less osteoporosis, less postpartum
depression, and faster postpartum weight loss. While you
may think of breastfeeding as all giving, giving, giving—
especially on those marathon days when your baby wants
to breastfeed all day and night—there is actually a mutual
give-and-take to the breastfeeding relationship.

   You give your baby the best nutritional start, and your
baby gives something back to you in return. Every time
you breastfeed, your mothering hormones soar. This
enables you to relax and get to know your baby. These hor-

mones appear to be the biochemical basis of the term "mother's intuition."

Introvert vs. Extrovert

Q *My baby's only a month old, but is there anything about her behavior now that could hint at what her personality may be?*

A You can get a hint of your baby's personality within a few days to weeks after birth. Newborns with an easy or laid-back personality usually don't cry as much if their needs are not immediately attended to. They tend to eat and sleep at more predictable times and in general seem less demanding. The other type of personality that you can spot early is a fascinating little character we have dubbed the "high-need" baby.

Some experts have labeled high-need babies inaccurately as colicky babies. They seem to be constantly-in-arms-and-at-breast infants who are content as long as they are held but fuss when they are put down. Some babies adjust to life outside the womb; high-need babies fuss to fit. While it's incorrect to give a tiny baby a permanent personality tag, infants do show their basic temperaments early on.

"Temperament" describes the basic emotional line of your baby. How your baby expresses her unique mind is through her personality. What kind of person your child becomes depends on her inborn temperament (nature) and your responses to it (nurture). Temperament is not good or bad; it's simply how your baby is. There will be times your typically fussy baby is content or your laid-back baby demands to be picked up.

It's important to fully understand the temperament not only of your baby but of yourself as well. Parent and baby need to find a way to fit. This little word so economically describes the relationship between baby and parent. Some parents fit together more easily, but many mothers and fathers and their babies have to make a few adjustments along the way to improve the fit. If your baby has high needs and a personality that demands that those needs be met, and you are a person who loves to be in control with a smooth, predictable routine, you and your baby will have to do some adjusting. Because babies and parents have different personalities, one style of parenting does not fit all families.

The goal of parenting a high-need baby is to allow baby and parent to shape each other's behavior so that the personalities mesh rather than clash. Eventually you will bring out the best in each other.

☙

Newborn Feeding Routines

Q   *How much should a newborn baby be fed? Should I schedule my baby's feedings? If so, what sort of schedule should I follow? And how will I know she's getting enough to eat?*

A We prefer to use the term "routine" rather than "schedule," which has a rigid ring to it. The term "routine" implies an arrangement that meets the nutritional needs of the infant while at the same time fits somewhat into the daily routine of the caregiver. Newborns should not be fed on a rigid three- to four-hour schedule, because they go through periodic growth spurts. It's only natural for a baby to eat more food during these growth periods. Also, feeding routines depend on an infant's temperament. Some easy-temperament infants adapt quickly to a predictable routine and feed every three hours. During growth spurts, they may feed every two hours, even around the clock.

How quickly baby develops a feeding routine also depends on whether baby is fed by breast or bottle. Breast-fed babies feed more frequently because breast milk is more easily and quickly digested and empties from the tummy faster. Because formula is slower to digest and infants feel full longer, formula-fed infants can often adapt to an every-three-hours feeding routine.

With breastfeeding you can't count ounces, so it's more challenging to know how much baby is getting. Signs that your newborn is getting enough breast milk are:

- *Number of wet diapers.* A baby who is getting enough milk will have four to six wet diapers a day by the fourth day after birth (six to eight diapers if you're using cloth, which hold less). To learn what a wet diaper feels like, put 2 tablespoons of water on a clean diaper. Cloth diapers will be more noticeably wet than superabsorbent disposable diapers. It may be easier to judge the wetness of a disposable by comparing its weight to a dry diaper than by feeling the surface of the diaper. After the first month or so, your baby's wet diapers will be even wetter (the equivalent of 4 to 6 tablespoons of water).

- *Color of urine.* A baby who is getting enough milk to keep him adequately hydrated will have pale or nearly clear urine. If the urine is darker, apple juice–colored (after the first four days), your baby is not getting enough milk. If your baby is not getting sufficient amounts of milk, you may also notice a "brick dust" residue on the diaper. This is a result of urate crystals from overly concentrated urine (a normal finding in the first few days), which should disappear after you increase baby's milk intake. Talk to your doctor to determine if your baby is getting enough milk during the time he is learning to breastfeed better.

- *Number and nature of bowel movements.* A baby who is getting enough milk will have many stools. In the first few days, infants' stools gradually change from the sticky, black meconium stools to green, then brown. Within a day or two of mother's milk "coming in," the stools become "milk stools." These are yellow or mustard-colored, seedy, and the consistency of cottage cheese. Between weeks one and four, breastfed babies who are getting enough hindmilk—the richer, high-calorie milk—will produce at least two to three yellow, seedy stools a day. Because breast milk is a natural laxative, some breastfed babies produce a stool with each feeding, which is a good sign that baby is getting ample milk. When a baby has only two or three bowel movements a day, expect to see a substantial amount in the diaper—more than just a stain.

After the first month or two, as the gut matures, the frequency of bowel movements decreases. At this stage, your baby may normally have only one bowel movement a day. Some babies have one bowel movement every three to four days but are still getting enough milk. During this period, you will notice other signs of adequate growth, such as weight gain.

While urine output tells you that baby is getting a sufficient quantity of fluid from the milk, stool output tells you about the quality of the milk. Baby's stools can let you know if she is nursing long enough and well enough to trigger the mother's milk-ejection reflex, which brings the creamier, high-calorie hindmilk. When a week-old baby is not producing sufficient stools, it's time to take a close look at whether baby is sucking correctly (see the discussion of latch-on, below).

✍

Avoiding Latch-On Problems

Q *I want to breastfeed my new baby, but I don't think I can take dealing with the kind of latch-on problems my sister had with her baby. What should I do to ensure a smooth start when my baby comes?*

A Breastfeeding works, or the human race would not exist. Yet the early weeks of breastfeeding are not as easy as is usually portrayed. Once you get through those early weeks, your baby will settle down to a comfortable breastfeeding relationship. In our thirty years of helping mothers and babies enjoy breastfeeding, we have noticed that mothers who get the right start at breastfeeding are more likely to enjoy this relationship. Here are seven starter tips we have found helpful:

1. Join La Leche League International (LLLI). This international volunteer organization presents information and support to women who breastfeed their babies and can be a valuable parenting support group while you are breastfeeding your baby.

2. Choose supportive friends. Surround yourself with friends who inspire confidence and affirm your choices in parenting and breastfeeding. Shun negative advisers, especially those who preach, "Maybe you don't have enough milk . . ." Don't let anyone sabotage your breastfeeding relationship, especially in those early weeks of getting started.

3. Take a breastfeeding class. The hospital where you plan to birth your baby is likely to offer breastfeeding classes.

4. Contact a professional lactation consultant. Contact a lactation consultant before the birth to schedule a hands-on demonstration of proper positioning and latch-on the day your baby is born.

5. Teach baby efficient latch-on. The most important key to successful breastfeeding is teaching your baby to latch on properly as she sucks from your breast. In this way your baby will get more milk and you will experience fewer breastfeeding problems, such as sore nipples, engorgement, and the feeling of having an inadequate milk supply. In a nutshell, get baby to open her mouth as wide as possible so that her lips are positioned high on your areola (babies suck areolas, not nipples!). Press down on her chin and pull out her lower lip (a technique we dubbed the "lower lip flip") to get baby to open her mouth wider and comfortably position her lower lip. Don't let her pucker her lips or put a tight mouth around your nipples—this the most common cause of poor latch-on.

6. Think positively. Have confidence that your body will work for you to deliver breast milk to your baby.

7. Make a commitment to a thirty-day trial. Remember, for centuries mothers have breastfed their babies through famines, wars, and a variety of less-than-ideal situations. In essence, once you are convinced of the value of breastfeeding, you will find a way to make it successful. The first couple of weeks are usually the most challenging, as baby is learning proper latch-on and you're getting used to being a mother. As a helpful reminder to get the right start in breastfeeding your baby, remember these "five C's": camaraderie, class, consultants, confidence, and commitment.

☙

Saving Breast Milk

Q *How long does breast milk keep when frozen, refrigerated, and at room temperature?*

A In the early weeks and months of breastfeeding, it helps to build a milk bank for circumstances that would briefly prevent you from breastfeeding, such as illnesses, being away from your baby at feeding time, or any other situation in which you may need your stored milk. Be sure to use clean containers, and wash your hands with soap and water before expressing or pumping milk.

Follow safe guidelines for storing breast milk. Breast milk can be safely kept at room temperature (66° to 72° F) for four to ten hours. It can be kept in a refrigerator for eight days, in a freezer compartment inside a refrigerator for two weeks, and in a separate deep-freeze unit for at least six months. Unused previously frozen breast milk that has been thawed can be safely kept in the refrigerator for up to twenty-four hours. Freshly collected breast milk that has been kept in the refrigerator for eight days but not used can be safely transferred to the freezer. Any breast milk that remains in a bottle after a feeding should be used for the next feeding but not kept thereafter. Bacteria from baby's mouth can enter the milk during the feeding, and if the milk sits too long, this can cause contamination. You can get plastic containers specifically made to hold human milk from La Leche League International or from your breast pump distributor.

⳼

A Newborn's Fingernails

Q *When is it okay to cut a newborn's fingernails for the first time? The hospital made it sound like I shouldn't cut them right away. My sister bit off her newborn's nails. Is that a good practice?*

A Although many newborns enter the world with fingernails long enough to scratch their adorable little faces, the hospital staff usually refuse to cut infants' fingernails, mainly for legal reasons in the event that a nurse clipped too deeply and cut a baby's finger. Instead, they ask parents to cut their baby's fingernails the day after leaving the hospital.

It's okay to bite off your newborn's nails, but there's an easier way. Wait until your baby is in a deep sleep, recognized by the limp-limb sign, when her limbs dangle limply at her side. Then cut her nails with a pair of nail clippers, preferably a set designed for babies.

To avoid snipping the fingertip skin as you clip the nail, depress the finger pad away from the nail as you cut. As a beginning nail cutter, have your spouse hold baby's hand while you manipulate the finger and the nail clipper. After a while you will be able to trim baby's nails by yourself.

Don't feel like a child abuser if you accidentally draw a few drops of blood. Every parent will accidentally go too deep at one time or another. A nail that was clipped too closely seldom gets infected, though it would be wise to apply an antibiotic ointment to the damaged skin for a few days afterward.

Newborn nails are soft and cut easily, but they grow quickly, so try to keep them trimmed as close as you possibly can. Toenails don't grow as fast and tend to be harder to get at without cutting baby. Don't cut them as often as you do the fingernails.

❧

Circumcision

Q *Do you consider circumcision a necessary procedure? Are there any health advantages? I read somewhere that the benefits aren't as great as was once thought.*

A No part of an infant's body has stirred as much debate as the foreskin. Even the American Academy of Pediatrics (AAP) has gone back and forth on this issue. In 1989, prompted by research that showed a link between circumcision and urinary tract infections (UTIs) and sexually transmitted diseases, the AAP concluded that the procedure did have medical benefits and advantages as well as risks. In 1999 the AAP reversed its recommendation, stating that the benefits of circumcision are not significant enough to recommend it as a routine procedure. The consensus among pediatricians is that there is no universal medical reason for routine circumcision.

While a few studies have suggested that the risk of UTIs is higher in uncircumcised boys than in boys who are circumcised, these studies have been statistical in nature. The foreskin hasn't been proven to be the cause of an increased occurrence of UTIs. Besides, UTIs are rare in males, circumcised or not. Research indicates that during the first year of life an uncircumcised male infant has at most a 1 in 100 chance of developing a UTI, while a circumcised male has about a 1 in 1,000 chance.

Research has also found that the risk of an uncircumcised man developing penile cancer is more than three times that of a circumcised man. However, penile cancer is extremely rare, with only nine to ten cases diagnosed per one million men each year. Studies have also suggested that circumcised men may be at a reduced risk for developing syphilis and HIV infections, but behavioral factors are the most important determinant of whether a man is at risk of contracting a sexually transmitted disease.

That being the case, the question of whether to circumcise your son is largely a personal decision. And while circumcision was once considered a routine procedure for newborn males in the United States, more and more parents are now questioning its necessity.

Here are some facts to consider when deciding whether or not to circumcise your baby:

- *Surgical risks*. Circumcision is usually a very safe surgical procedure. Yet, as with any surgical procedure, there is the rare problem of bleeding, infection, or injury to the penis.
- *Pain*. The circumcision procedure hurts. The myth that newborns do not feel pain during the circumcision came from the fact that newborns sometimes withdraw into a deep sleep toward the end of the operation. But this is actually a retreat mechanism, a withdrawal reaction to overwhelming pain. Studies have since shown that during unanesthetized circumcision, stress hormones rise, the heart rate speeds up, and the oxygen content of the baby's blood diminishes. The AAP's recommendation is that if parents decide to circumcise their infant, pain relief must be provided.

  Most doctors today perform circumcision using a local anesthetic. If you choose to circumcise your infant, insist that it be done under local anesthesia. The most common and effective method is called a dorsal penile nerve block, in which a few drops of Xylocaine (similar to the anesthetic your dentist uses) are injected into the nerves on each side of the penis. This seldom relieves all the pain of circumcision, but in most cases it significantly reduces it.
- *Rationale*. Having a baby circumcised just so he won't feel different from his friends isn't a good enough reason to go ahead with the procedure. The percentage of intact males has risen steadily in recent years and is probably

about fifty-fifty nationwide by now. Locker-room comparisons and the "like father, like son" feeling are outdated—few fathers and sons compare foreskins. Some parents have their sons circumcised for religious or cultural reasons.

The circumcision debate is likely to continue for years, even as routine circumcision becomes a thing of the past. It's up to each family to decide what is right for their child.

ᔕ

Baby Sneezes

Q *My newborn appears to sneeze a lot. Could it be that she's caught a cold already?*

A While your baby's sneezing could be a cold, it's more likely that she's reacting to something either in the air or stuck in her nasal passages. Newborns are nose breathers and don't breathe very well through their mouths. Sneezing is how they clear congested airways.

If your baby isn't able to clear her nose and is forced to breathe through her mouth, she's likely to get very upset. If this is the case, you need to "hose the nose." You can do this by spritzing the inside of her nostrils with a few drops of saline, available over the counter in a small squirt bottle. Then vacuum her nasal secretions out with a nasal aspirator, a gadget affectionately dubbed a "snot snatcher" by veteran parents in our practice. Common signs that it's time to clear the nose include a tendency to pull off the breast or bottle to catch her breath or more frequent awakenings.

Work to shield your baby from common airborne allergens, such as cigarette smoke, animal dander, and dust. Don't allow smoking in the same house as baby. Also, avoid paint and gasoline fumes, aerosols, perfumes, and hair sprays. Notify your doctor if your newborn is feverish, lethargic, pale, or just appears sick.

Be particularly vigilant in allergy-proofing baby's sleeping environment:

- Remove dust collectors, like stuffed animals and fuzzy toys.
- Use a HEPA-type air filter in your infant's bedroom to remove pollens and dust mites. HEPA filters are efficient in filtering out almost 100 percent of airborne allergens and danders.
- Close your baby's bedroom window at night to block pollens from nearby plants and trees.
- Wash her hair before bedtime to remove pollens that may have collected during the day.

⌒

Learning the Language of a Newborn

Q *How can I differentiate my baby's "I need something now" screaming from normal newborn fussing?*

A A baby's cry is a baby's language, defined for the survival of baby and the development of the parent. Above all, avoid the "let baby cry it out" crowd! This bad baby advice only weakens the trust your baby has in you. It also desensitizes you to the cues of your infant and keeps you from learning how to read your baby's earliest language.

In the early weeks you won't always know how to read your baby's cry. Is she hungry, restless, or uncomfortable and needing some immediate nurturing? Or is she just blowing off a little steam and will comfort herself if left alone for a few minutes? These are "cry by cry" reads, which time and experience will help you to decode.

The best rule of thumb on infant crying is that in the early weeks respond promptly to your child's cry. Don't go through the mental gymnastics of thinking you will spoil her if you pick her up every time she cries. After you and your baby have rehearsed this on-cue response hundreds of times in the early months, you will learn to tell the difference between a "red-alert" cry that needs immediate attention and a cry to which you can delay your response for a while in the hope baby can soothe herself. Once you develop your maternal sensitivity to your infant's cries, you will intuitively know which ones need an immediate response.

In general, a cry of pain begins suddenly, reaches a high pitch quickly, and seems to stay at that high pitch for a while. Pain cries are shrill and shrieking. Your baby's mouth is wide open as if saying ouch. Her jaws quiver, her face grimaces, her fists are clenched, and her legs are drawn up and her whole body language shouts, "I hurt, help me!" Sometimes infants with frantic or pain cries will hold their breath for ten to fifteen seconds (which seems like an eternity). Also, pain cries continue for a bit after baby is picked up. Normal newborn fussing tends to quick-

ly subside once baby is picked up. Cries arising from pain
are often frustratingly inconsolable.

Please note that mothers are biologically wired to
respond to their infants' cries. The advice to let your baby
cry it out is biologically incorrect. If you and your baby
were wired up to some physiological sensors, whenever
your baby cried, the blood flow to your breasts would actually increase. This is because you have a biological urge to
pick up and comfort your baby—not to ignore her cries.

✍

Evaluating Breastfeeding

Q *Are there signs I can notice or feel that my breasts
are producing enough milk for my baby? I'm not a large-
breasted mom!*

A While you breastfeed your baby, look for these
breast signs that your baby is getting enough milk:

- Your breasts will feel fuller before feeding and softer
  after a feeding. Changes in fullness will be less noticeable when baby is older and your breasts become more
  efficient at producing the exact amount of milk your
  baby needs.
- A milk-ejection reflex will happen a few minutes after
  the feeding begins. If you don't feel any sensation in
  your breasts, watch your baby. His sucking will intensify, and you'll hear more frequent swallowing when the
  milk-ejection reflex increases the milk flow.

- A few drops of milk will leak from the sides of baby's mouth.
- Baby will suck vigorously and swallow after every one or two sucks. Your baby will seem content during and after a feeding and may drift contentedly off to sleep.

⁊

Weight Gain in Newborns

Q *My first baby weighed more than 7 pounds when she was born. When we were leaving the hospital, the nurse told us she had lost 3 ounces. I worried that something was wrong. Now I'm expecting our second child. Is there anything I can do to prevent baby's weight loss after birth?*

A Your doctor will check your newborn's weight a few days after you leave the hospital and perhaps again a week or two later. Most infants, whether breastfed or bottlefed, will lose an average of 5 to 7 percent of their birth weight in the first days of life due to the loss of excess fluid. How much they lose depends on their plumpness and individual variations in fluid retention as well as on how well they are nursing.

When mothers and babies share an uncomplicated birth, babies feed frequently and learn to latch on to the breast so they can suck efficiently. Babies who get off to a slow start at breastfeeding (either because of a medical complication or problems with latch-on) tend to lose more weight. Babies who are getting adequate amounts of milk weigh within 1 or 2 ounces of their birth weight at their one-week checkup. Some infants take a couple of weeks to regain their birth weight, especially if they lose a lot initially.

When you are discharged from the hospital, remember to ask the nurse to give you baby's weight. Your doctor will want to know this number at your baby's first checkup, since weight gain is measured from baby's lowest weight, not from the birth weight. After regaining his birth weight, the average infant gains 4 to 7 ounces a week, or a minimum of 1 pound a month. Some babies gain weight quickly in the first months after birth; others gain more slowly but are still within the normal range.

◯⁓

A Newborn's Nervous System

Q *My newborn's movements seem really jerky and abrupt. Is this normal?*

A In the first few months, because baby's nervous system is immature, you may notice normal chin quivers, twitches of arms and legs, and lip twitches while baby is sleeping (dubbed "sleep grins"). Also, when you play with baby's arms and legs, you will often notice they spring back with jerky movements. As your baby's nervous system matures, these quivers, twitches, and jerky involuntary muscle movements will subside.

⁊⁊

Eye Discharge

Q *I discovered some odd-looking matter coming out of my newborn's eyes. What is it, and how do I get rid of it?*

A   The discharge you are noticing from your baby's eyes is caused by blocked tear ducts. Sometimes debris collects in the tiny canals (tear ducts) that drain tears from the eyes to the nose, causing the tears to accumulate in the nasal corners of the eyes. If these tears do not drain properly, the ducts often become infected. When the tear ducts open more widely, this eye drainage problem should subside—usually by six months of age.

To unclog your baby's tear ducts gently massage the nasal corner of your baby's eye where the discharge is occurring. You will oftentimes feel a tiny bump in this area where the tear duct is located. With the tip of your well-scrubbed, short-nailed pinkie finger, massage the tear duct about six times several times a day; get into the habit of doing it before each diaper change. If the yellowish discharge persists, the tears may require an antibiotic eye ointment available by prescription from your baby's doctor. If the tear ducts don't open by themselves by nine to twelve months, it's sometimes necessary for an eye doctor to open them by inserting a tiny wire into the duct, a procedure called tear-duct probing. This is done under light anesthesia either as an office procedure or outpatient surgery.

∽

Bathing a Baby

Q *Am I a bad mom if I bathe my newborn only twice a week? It's just such a production to wash him.*

A Newborns really don't need a daily bath. Except for his diaper area, there is very little on baby's body that gets dirty. Most new mothers suffer from what we call the "mother cat syndrome," overwashing their newborns as an instinct of good mothering.

A total body bath once or twice a week is plenty. The areas that need the most bathing are the skin folds of the neck, under the arms, and in the groin or diaper area. As with feeding, consider bathing your baby a social interaction. Here are some safe baby-bathing tips we have enjoyed:

- *Wear "kid gloves."* Wear a pair of old white gloves and rub a little mild baby soap on them. You have an instant washcloth that automatically shapes itself to baby's body and reduces the slipperiness of bare hands on soapy skin.
- *Pat, don't rub, the skin with the washcloth and blot skin dry with a towel.* Vigorous scrubbing irritates a newborn's sensitive skin. A newborn's skin is sensitive to some soaps, so use soap only on areas that are caked with secretions, such as oil or sweat behind the ears, in the neck folds, and in the creases of the groin.
- *When first using soap, test it on a small part of the body.*

If baby's skin reddens or gets dry and flaky on that area, the soap is too strong. Babies usually tolerate a mild soap, such as Dove. Since soap robs the skin of its natural oils, use a mild soap and use it sparingly, no more than a couple times a week. Wash off the soap as soon as possible and rinse the area well.

- *Shampoo the scalp with a mild shampoo no more than once a week.* Overuse can irritate the scalp.
- *Avoid powder and oils.* Your baby's skin is naturally rich in oil. If inhaled, powder or fragrances may irritate baby's sensitive nasal passages.
- *If baby protests a bath, enjoy a bath for two.* Fill the tub to breast level and sit yourself in the tub first. Have someone hand baby to you and hold your baby close to you. Nurse her for a while. You can then bathe baby while you relax in the tub yourself. If your baby has a water phobia, you may convince her she's just getting a wet massage instead of a bath.

Newborn Shots and Tests

Q *What sort of shots and tests can I expect my baby to have at birth and during the early months?*

A In the hospital and during the early months you can expect the following preventive medicine for your baby:

Vitamin K Shot and Eye Ointment

Because baby may be temporarily deficient in vitamin K immediately after birth, she is given an injection of this vitamin. Vitamin K promotes normal blood clotting and reduces the risk of abnormal bleeding. Usually the nurse will give this shot along with an antibiotic eye ointment used to protect your newborn against germs that may have entered her eyes during passage through the birth canal. You may request that the nurse delay these procedures for a few hours until you and your newborn have had a chance to begin bonding.

Vaccines

Some newborns receive the hepatitis B vaccine within the first day or two after birth while still in the hospital. This is to make sure they get at least one of the series of three vaccine shots they are supposed to receive but sometimes don't if parents neglect the medical follow-up.

Because hepatitis B is transmitted by sexual contact or blood products, there is seldom a medical reason to give a newborn this shot. Unless there is a medical reason, I advise against giving newborns this shot because the occasional newborn will react to the vaccine with fever and lethargy, causing alarm and unnecessary medical tests for possible newborn infection. Except in special circumstances, you can safely defer giving this vaccine to your newborn until a routine office visit with your baby's doctor a few months later.

Most "baby shots" begin on baby's two-month visit. The vaccines routinely given at this visit are DPT (diphtheria, pertussis, tetanus) and HIB (the hemophilus influenza B), which is a vaccine against the germ that causes such serious infections as meningitis and pneumonia. You can expect your baby to get two or three immunizations (DPT, HIB, injectable polio, and hepatitis B) at two, four, and six months of age.

Newborn Screening Tests

Before you leave the hospital with your baby, a few drops of blood are taken from your baby's heel to test for rare diseases that are treatable if detected early. These diseases include:

- *Hypothyroidism.* This condition occurs in one out of every five thousand infants, and if undetected and untreated may cause mental retardation. If it is detected and treated early, babies can develop normally.
- *Phenylketonuria (PKU).* This rare disease occurs in only one out of fifteen thousand infants. If this condition continues untreated, it can result in brain damage. If it is detected by a special newborn screening test and treated early, the child can develop normally with a special diet.
- *Galactosemia.* This extremely rare condition occurs in one out of sixty thousand infants. With galactosemia, an enzyme deficiency allows harmful substances to build up in baby's blood and damage vital tissues. If left untreated it is fatal. This condition is treatable by a special diet.

Blood Type

Unless specifically ordered by a doctor, many hospitals do not routinely check a newborn's blood type. Still, a sample of your baby's umbilical cord blood is routinely taken in case you or the doctor want to know your baby's blood type and Rh factor.

✑

What Your Baby Sees and Hears

Q *My son is fifteen days old, and I'm curious about his ability to see and hear. What can I do with my baby that would have meaning to him?*

A Newborns are engaged by certain sights and sounds. Research has shown that the human face—especially a familiar one—is a particularly riveting attention-holder. Another favorite eye-catcher is light-and-dark contrast, such as black-and-white drawings of a face or contrasting patterns. Checkerboards, stripes, and bull's-eyes are favorite patterns for crib mobiles. Because of the preference for light-and-dark contrast, babies often pay close attention to a male face with a beard or a mustache.

To capture your little one's attention, sit your baby on your lap or hold him upright; babies are more visually attentive when upright than when lying down. Your baby will be most visually engaged in the state of quiet alertness, with eyes fully open and body calm. Babies love exaggerated facial gestures, such as wide-open mouth and eyes. This is why a mother's animated face and the classic cartoon characters are time-honored favorites.

To determine the distance at which your baby sees best, hold him 10 inches from your face and make direct eye contact. As you move your little one closer and farther from this intimate space, notice where he breaks the visual connection and loses interest when your image becomes hazy.

Studies show that babies understand a great deal, even in the early months. Video analysis of mother-baby interaction reveals that newborns move their heads and bodies in synchrony with Mom's speech, as if dancing in time to the rhythm of her voice. More of your messages are getting through to your baby than you realize.

Sometimes newborns prefer their mother's high-pitched voice; at other times they like Dad's lower, more monotonous tones, which are reminiscent of the sounds heard from the womb. Babies also like music with a womblike beat, preferring the predictable rising and falling rhythms of classical music to the disorderly rhythms of rock and roll. To hold your baby's auditory attention, develop eye contact before you begin talking. Babies often become confused if they can't see who's talking to them.

Moms are naturals when it comes to communicating with infants, instinctively adopting the upbeat tones and facial gestures of motherese, as explained on pages 30–31. How you speak to your baby depends upon the reaction you want from him. High-pitched, exaggerated, and animated speech tends to rev up baby during playtime. To wind baby down for a nap or at bedtime, sing or hum a lullaby or other monotonous tune. "Ol' Man River" is a favorite with dads because it's low and droning and easy to sing.

The visual and auditory stimulation you provide while interacting with your infant not only encourages development but also increases the connection you have with your little one.

⊘

Newborn Breast Swelling

Q *My three-week-old grandson has developed a pea-size lump under his nipple. What could this be?*

A The pea-size lump under your grandson's nipple is common in newborns. This swelling is normal breast tissue that has been stimulated to grow by the maternal hormones that passed into his bloodstream from his mother during pregnancy. Curiously, some newborns even produce a few drops of milk from their nipples due to the same hormonal process. The swellings are painless and harmless, and they generally subside within a couple of months.

⊘

Newborn Noisy Breathing

Q *My newborn's breathing seems really uneven and noisy. Sometimes she grunts and squeaks and sounds congested. Is this something that I should bring up with my doctor?*

A Welcome to the world of noisy children. Your previously quiet home now has a lot of background "music" that begins with normal newborn noises. Newborns sneeze, sputter, and gurgle. Not only do newborns breathe noisily, but they breathe irregularly. Newborns tend to take frequent short breaths interspersed with an occasional deep sigh. Then there may be a five- to ten-second period (which seems like an eternity) when your newborn holds her breath. This normal pattern is called periodic breathing.

By two to three months of age your baby's breathing becomes more regular but still may be noisy. Sometime during the second month expect more noisy breathing that may sound like baby's first cold but usually is not. You may even feel a rattling in your baby's chest when you put your hand on her back. These are normal sounds caused by the pooling of saliva in the back of the throat. When air passes through this puddle it vibrates and produces rattling sounds. If your baby's noisy breathing is simply due to this normal development, she'll sound congested but won't experience any discomfort. As long as she feeds and sleeps well, there's no need for concern about the congestion. Once your baby learns to swallow the excess pre-teething saliva, these breathing noises will subside.

On the other hand, your daughter may be allergic to something in her immediate sleeping environment—probably dust collectors, such as fuzzy toys. Do some detective work to identify and remove dust collectors from the area where she sleeps. It is also possible that your baby's noisy breathing is caused by an inflammation of the vocal cords left over from suctioning procedures at birth. If this is the case, inhalations will be noticeably noisier than exhalations, and the sound will be consistent with each breath. The random grunts and squeaks you describe sound like normal breathing noises. Whatever the cause, your baby is likely to outgrow these sound effects within the next couple of months. During that time, she'll learn to swallow her excess saliva, and any vocal-cord inflammation will gradually heal—and, of course, you will have allergy-proofed her sleeping environment.

Babies need a clear nose to breathe and do not comfortably switch from nose to mouth breathing if the nasal passages are plugged. If your baby seems to be nasally congested, flush her nose with saltwater nose drops. This solution, available over the counter at your pharmacy, comes in a tiny squirt bottle. You can also make your own nose drops by dissolving a pinch of salt (no more than ¼ teaspoon) in an 8-ounce glass of warm tap water. Then use a plastic eyedropper to squirt a few drops into each nostril and gently suction the nose clear using a nasal aspirator. We call this technique "hosing the nose."

We remember how noisily our babies breathed during the first few months. Here are some favorite baby sounds and the labels parents have attached to them:

- *Gurgle:* caused by air passing through pooled saliva in the back of the mouth
- *Snurgle:* a gurgle accompanied by nasal congestion (a combination of a snort and a gurgle)
- *Blurp:* a burp that passes through mucus in the mouth or throat
- *Burble:* a burp accompanied by bubbles

Normal breathing may also take on a purring quality when air and saliva compete for the same space. During sleep, the already narrow breathing passages relax and become even narrower, causing each breath to take on a musical, grunting, or sighing quality. And, of course, who can forget those delightful birdlike chirps and squeaks?

Enjoy these precious baby sounds; they won't last long!

Burping a Baby

Q   *How often should I burp my baby? Only after each feeding? Should I interrupt a feeding to burp him if he's eating a great deal? I've read that you should burp after every ounce of formula. Is that true?*

A   Some babies are born air swallowers and need to be burped a lot; others aren't. Gulpers tend to be air swallowers and need frequent and effective burping; slower feeders tend to need less burping. Breastfed infants tend to swallow less air because they can control the flow of milk more easily than bottlefed babies can. If your baby is comfortable after feeding and does not appear bloated or colicky, then you don't need to worry if you're not able to get up a burp.

In general, try to burp your baby after each feeding. Persist for a few minutes and if no burp appears, relax. Here are some ways you can reduce the amount of air your baby swallows:

• Feed your baby in an upright position.
• Make sure your breastfeeding infant forms a tight seal during latch-on (see page 57).

• Keep your infant upright and quiet for twenty to thirty minutes after feeding to allow air to settle to the top of his stomach.

Don't feel you have failed Infant Care 101 if you don't manage to bring up a burp at every feeding. Oftentimes babies don't need to burp after a small snack-type feeding. After a big meal, it's usually worth putting in some patient effort until your baby burps.

While there are many burping positions, they all have in common an upright (30- to 45-degree-angle) position and pressure placed on baby's tummy. The most effective burping position is the over-the-hand burp. Sit baby on your lap facing away from you, and place the heel of your hand against her tummy, with her chin resting on the top of your hand. Lean baby forward, resting most of her weight against the heel of your hand to provide pressure on her tummy, and pat her on the back to get up the air bubbles. Or drape baby over your shoulder to let your shoulder press against her tummy and then rub her back. Be sure you have a cloth over your shoulder to catch the inevitable spit-up.

At nighttime, burping is often not necessary. Babies swallow less air because they feed more slowly and do not take in as much at night. If a trapped air bubble seems to be causing some abdominal pain at night, drape baby over your hip as you lie on your side. This will get the air up more easily and get you and baby back to sleep more quickly.

✑

Warming Breast Milk

Q *My wife (a family practitioner) insists that I shouldn't microwave breast milk because "it screws up the proteins or something." I think she's misinterpreted the common admonition not to microwave baby's food or drink because of the potential uneven heating and possibility of burning baby. Who's right?*

A We advise against microwaving breast milk. Valuable components of the milk are destroyed if it's heated over 130° F. Heating of any type, especially microwaving, does alter the proteins. Whether or not it changes their nutritional value or health benefits to the body is unknown.

A major concern about microwaving breast milk is that it kills the living white cells. In some cultures, breast milk is known as white blood, since it contains millions of immune-fighting proteins and living white blood cells. And it's true that microwaving heats liquids unevenly, causing hot spots in the milk (whether formula, cow's milk, or breast milk) that could burn baby.

☙

Getting to a Predictable Routine

Q *When can I expect my baby to settle into a routine of some sort? I haven't been able to sleep for a straight two-hour stretch since my baby was born a month ago. The house is a mess, my hair is a disaster, and most of my shirts are stained with substances that either came out of or were meant to go into my newborn. Is raising a newborn this hard for everyone?*

A Most mothers describe life with a new baby as all-consuming. But how consuming an infant is really depends a lot on the baby's temperament. Certain babies—we dub them "high-need" babies—require a higher-than-normal level of care. It's almost like the high-need baby at birth comes out and says, "Hi, Mom and Dad. You've been blessed with an above-average baby, and I need above-average parenting. If you give it to me, we'll get along fine. If you don't, we're gong to have a bit of trouble along the road."

These babies have a higher-than-average need to be held. They don't schedule easily. They often wake up frequently for night feedings. These are bright and energetic yet exhausting infants. High-need babies, though challenging, often grow up to be bright and interesting children.

Some infants adjust to life after birth more easily than others. Easy or laid-back infants adjust to a consistent caregiving routine, while others remain unpredictable for the first six months. That's why it's important to develop a style of caregiving that lets you also enjoy living with your child. Feeling exhausted and overwhelmed leaves Mom burned out. Mothers are usually naturally giving persons, so it's easy to keep giving and giving until you totally give out. With one of our high-need babies, I remember Martha saying, "My baby needs me so much that I don't have time to take a shower." Later that day I put a sign on the bathroom mirror that read: "Each day remember what our baby needs most—a happy, rested mother."

Even though it seems like all you do during the early months is give and give, your newborn is giving something to you, too: teaching you the delicate art of parenting. Granted, there will be days when you feel like you are getting nothing done. But you *are* getting something done! You are raising a precious human being.

As far as sleeping through the night, realistically, the only tiny infant who really sleeps through the night is the one in a book (or your best friend's baby!). It's a fact that newborns have tiny tummies and need to be fed frequently. Studies have shown that infants do not reach five-hour stretches of sleep until around six months. When an infant starts sleeping in longer stretches depends mostly on individual temperament.

To help ease your baby into a more predictable routine so that you can enjoy living with one another, try the following suggestions:

- *Raise a "sling baby."* Wearing your baby in a sling around the house or even out of the house while you are shopping calms baby and allows you to get things done yet still be close to your infant.
- *Nap when baby naps.* It's important to resist the temptation to get something done while baby is sleeping. You need a nap to recharge your energy as much as your infant does.

- *Get daily exercise.* Put baby in a sling and take a walk together. This is especially important for infants who are "P.M. fussers," those who seem to have an hour or so of fussy time toward the end of the day. We call this time "happy hour."
- *Hire help.* If possible, have someone come in and clean your house once a week.
- *Reserve time for yourself.* Tend to your grooming. When you feel good about yourself physically, the feeling will carry over to your emotional happiness as a mother. Your baby will sense your contentment.
- *Realize this stage is short-term.* Take consolation in the fact that this high-maintenance stage doesn't last forever. The time in your arms, at your breast, and even in your bed is a relatively short period in the total life of your child. But the memories of love and availability will last a lifetime.

⌒

Bellybutton Basics

Q *How soon after the umbilical cord stump falls off can I give my baby a bath?*

A If the site where the cord was attached is completely dry and there is no redness around the edges (usually by two weeks), it is safe to immerse your baby in a bath. The key is to avoid infection in the cord area. If there is pus draining at the base of the cord, it is unwise to immerse baby in a bath for fear of contaminating the water and spreading the infection. In this case, you should sponge-bathe baby until the cord falls off and the stump is healed.

✑

Characteristics of High-Need Babies

Q *My six-week-old craves being held all the time. When I try to put her down, she cries. My friend says that she's a "high-need" baby. What exactly does this term mean? How do I know if she is indeed this type of baby?*

A We developed this term after the birth of Hayden, one of our babies. Unlike our other children, she demanded our constant attention. During the day she wanted to be held often and to nurse frequently. At night the only place where she would sleep was in our bed, snuggled close to us.

Hayden didn't fit any of the usual labels. She really wasn't "fussy" or "difficult," since as long as we attended to her needs she was content. Nor could she be considered "colicky," as she didn't seem to be in pain.

After talking with parents in our pediatric practice who had similar children, the term "high-need" came to us. It underscores the idea that these babies simply need more— more touch, more understanding, more sensitivity, and more creative parenting.

How do you know if you have this type of baby? Here are the most common characteristics that mothers note in describing their high-need infants:

- *"He's super-sensitive."* High-need babies are acutely aware of their environment and easily bothered by changes in their routines. They startle easily during the day and settle poorly at night. This sensitivity enables them to form deep attachments to trusted and consistent caregivers, but don't expect them to readily accept strangers or baby-sitters. They have selective tastes and definite mind-sets.
- *"I just can't put her down."* Motion, not stillness, is a way of life for these babies. These are in-arms, at-breast babies who seldom accept much downtime in a crib.
- *"He's not a self-soother."* This baby is known for his inability to self-soothe. Parents confide, "He can't relax by himself." Mother's lap is his chair, Father's arms and chest his crib, Mother's breasts his pacifier. These babies are very choosy about inanimate mother substitutes, such as cuddlies and pacifiers, and often forcefully reject them.
- *"He's intense."* "He's in high gear all the time," observed a tired father. High-need babies put a lot of energy into what they do. They cry loudly, laugh delightedly, and are quick to protest if their "meals" are not served on time.
- *"She wants to nurse all the time."* Expect a feeding schedule to be foreign to this baby's mind-set. She will try to marathon breastfeed every two to three hours around the clock and enjoy long periods of comfort sucking. Not only do these babies feed more often, they suck longer. High-need babies are notoriously slow to wean and usually breastfeed into the second or third year.

- *"He awakens frequently."* "Why do high-need babies need more of everything but sleep?" groaned a tired mother. They awaken frequently during the night and seldom reward their parents with a much-needed long nap during the day. You may feel that your baby has an internal light bulb that cannot easily turn off.

- *"She is never satisfied and is always unpredictable."* Just as you figure out what your baby needs, expect a change of plans. As one exhausted mother put it, "Just when I think I have the game won, she ups the ante." One set of comforting measures works one day but fails the next.

- *"He is hyperactive, hypertonic."* While being held, these babies squirm until you find their favorite position for being held. During nursing, they often arch their backs. "There's no such thing as a still shot," remarked a photographer father of his high-need baby. While holding some high-need babies, you can feel their muscles tense.

- *"She is absolutely draining."* Besides putting their own energy into what they do, these babies use up their parents' energy, too. "He wears me out" is a frequent complaint.

- *"He is so uncuddly."* Whereas most babies melt into their parents' arms and mold into comfortable positions while being held, the uncuddly high-need baby arches his back, stiffens his arms and legs, and withdraws from intimate holding. Most tiny babies crave physical contact and settle when held tightly and swaddled; uncuddly babies are slower to soften into a comfortable nestle in their parents' arms. Eventually most do if the mother persists in her efforts to bond, offering baby a safe, firm holding place he can give in to.

- *"She is demanding."* Babies with high needs have high

standards—and an equally strong personality to get what they need. Watch two babies raise their arms as "pick me up" gestures to their parents. If parents miss the cue, the mellower baby may put her arms down and begin to satisfy herself in play. Not so with the high-need baby, who at the unacceptable thought that the parent missed her cue will howl and continue her demands until she is picked up.

Be prepared for this demanding personality trait to set you up as a target for destructive advice such as, "She's manipulating you." "Manipulating" may be a forerunner of the later label "strong-willed" as the baby gets older. But consider for a moment what would happen if the high-need child were not demanding. If baby had a strong need but did not have a strong temperament to persist until the need was met, perhaps that baby would not thrive to her full potential.

Exhausted parents often ask, "How long will these traits last, and what can we expect as he grows?" Don't be too quick to predict the person your child will become. Some difficult babies show a complete turnabout in personality later in childhood. But in general, the needs of these babies do not lessen; they only change.

While these early personality traits may sound somewhat negative and initially may cause parents to feel a bit discouraged, those who strive to meet their baby's needs usually adopt a different outlook. Soon they begin using more positive labels, such as "challenging," "interesting," and "bright" to describe their child. The "intense baby" may soon become the "creative child"; the "sensitive infant," the "compassionate child"; and the "little taker," the "little giver."

ॐ

Alcohol and Breastfeeding

Q *I have a four-week-old son whom I'm breastfeeding. I haven't had anything alcoholic to drink since I learned I was pregnant. Can I safely have a drink or two now, or do I need to wait until I stop breastfeeding?*

A Much of the confusion surrounding this topic stems from two myths about breastfeeding and alcohol that are being challenged today by scientific research:

1. Wine is good for relaxing the nursing mom.
2. Beer is good for increasing milk supply.

Several studies now suggest that these two bits of folklore should be replaced by these new troubling facts:

1. Alcohol enters breast milk very rapidly and in concentrations nearly equal to that found in the maternal blood.
2. Your infant may not be able to sufficiently detoxify this alcohol from his system.

Researchers have noted slower motor development in the babies of mothers who drank while breastfeeding and report that the lags increase the more the mother drank.

Besides the damage to baby's development, alcohol can actually make breastfeeding more difficult, turning the relaxation myth on its head. Alcohol has been shown to inhibit the milk-ejection reflex, with increased alcohol having an even greater effect. Research on animals also showed that alcohol inhibits milk production and may give the milk an unpleasant flavor.

You should refrain from alcohol completely during or just before the act of breastfeeding, though the occasional glass of wine or beer is unlikely to harm your baby. We recommend conservative moderation for as long as you are breastfeeding your baby.

✑

Sterilizing Baby Bottles

Q *My sister and I are debating whether baby bottles need to be sterilized. I say they do—for at least the first six months. My sister thinks sterilizing isn't necessary at all. Who's right?*

A   You are. It's important to sterilize a baby's bottles for at least the first six months to protect against food-borne infections. This is because milk and formula residue is hard to remove and serves as a fertile breeding ground for germs that can cause diarrhea. For babies severe diarrhea can be a serious condition because dehydration can happen so quickly in infancy.

Fortunately, sterilizing is quite simple. A dishwasher with a water temperature of at least 180° F will adequately clean and sterilize bottles and their accessories. If your sister doesn't have a dishwasher, encourage her to try the following procedure after washing the equipment in hot, soapy water and rinsing it thoroughly: Pad the bottom of a large pot with a clean towel or dishcloth (to avoid sticking or breakage). Fill the pot with water and immerse open bottles, nipples, and other equipment in the pot (place bottles on their sides to be sure they get filled with the sterilizing water). Cover the pot and bring the water to a boil for ten minutes. The water and equipment should cool to room temperature while the pot is still covered. Finally, remove the bottles and nipples with tongs or spoons, place the bottles upside down on a clean towel with the nipples and caps alongside, and let the equipment dry. Make sure the place where bottles are stored is kept clean and dry.

⁊

Constipation from Iron-Fortified Formula

Q *Can the iron in infant formula cause constipation? My ten-week-old baby is constipated, although I give him up to an extra 4 ounces of water each day. We feed him Isomil (he became congested with a cow's-milk formula). If changing the formula doesn't help, what should I try next?*

A Opinion is divided on whether iron in infant formula can cause constipation in infants. Controlled studies performed by the late Dr. Frank Oski, Professor and Chairman of the Department of Pediatrics at Johns Hopkins Medical School, showed that iron-fortified formulas did not cause constipation any more than formulas without iron. But scientific research and mothers' firsthand observations sometimes clash. In our pediatric practice, a mother occasionally tells us she's absolutely certain that iron causes constipation.

Be aware that even if he is constipated, your baby does need an iron-fortified formula. Low-iron formulas simply don't provide adequate amounts of iron, resulting in anemia (low hemoglobin) between the ages of six and twelve months.

Here are some ways to relieve your baby's constipation:

- Continue giving him an extra 4 to 8 ounces of water a day.
- Experiment with different types of formula until you find one that is more intestines friendly. Soy formula tends to be constipating, so you might try a predigested formula, such as Alimentum or Nutramigen. But we recommend that you use these formulas as a last resort, since they are expensive and often unpalatable.
- Delay solid foods for several more months, since rice cereal and bananas (the usual starter foods) can be constipating.
- Feed your baby smaller amounts more frequently to aid digestion.
- Give your baby warm, daily baths while massaging his abdomen. This will help the stools move along through the intestines.
- If your baby strains during a bowel movement, insert half of an infant glycerin suppository into his rectum. These suppositories—available without prescription—resemble tiny rocketships, and you can use them every couple of days for a few weeks without your baby becoming dependent on them.

- Remember the four P's: prunes, pears, plums, and peaches. As he gets older, between seven and nine months, try adding prune or pear nectar and pureed prunes and pears to your baby's diet.

❦

Thrush and Other Fungal Infections

Q *My son was born with Listeria meningitis and spent twenty-one days in the hospital on antibiotics. He is doing fine now and doesn't seem to have any existing problems as a result of the infection. But last week we noticed whiteness on his tongue, which his doctor identified as thrush. Could my baby have had the thrush ever since he was taken off the antibiotics? And is he likely to encounter other infections or illnesses as a result of his medical history?*

A You are fortunate that the meningitis was caught early and treated and that you now have a normal, healthy baby. The antibiotics used to treat newborn meningitis need to be strong to treat the germs in the spinal fluid. These same antibiotics also kill the normal bacteria that inhabit the lining of the intestinal tract, beginning with the mouth.

Normally, the mouth and intestinal tract are coated with healthy bacteria that, in return for a warm place to live, contribute to the health of your baby's intestinal tract, manufacture vitamins, and battle harmful bacteria. The antibiotics your son received as an infant threw off this natural balance between helpful and harmful germs that line the intestinal tract, allowing the overgrowth of a fungus (or yeast) called thrush.

Thrush won't harm your baby, but it's a nuisance to deal with. If you are breastfeeding, you may also get this fungus infection on your nipples (they will redden, and you'll experience intense burning and itching). If this happens, put the thrush medicine your doctor prescribes for baby on your nipples several times a day.

Thrush is treated with prescription antifungal drops given three times a day for at least ten days. Paint the thrush medicine on your baby's tongue and all over the inside of his mouth, as your doctor prescribes. If you are formula feeding, it's helpful to mix a teaspoon of acidophilus powder in the bottle of formula once a day to enhance the growth of healthy nutrients and inhibit the growth of yeast. If you are breastfeeding, mix it in a little water, and administer it with a cup throughout the day. Secondary to the thrush, you may also notice a fungus-type diaper rash (a raised red ring around your baby's anus). An over-the-counter antifungal cream (Lotrimin) applied twice a day for a week should relieve this rash, but it may take several weeks for the thrush to disappear. After that, there is no reason why your infant should be more susceptible than any other infant to fungus infections.

᠅

A Newborn's Sleep-Wake Cycle

Q *Our three-week-old baby girl seems to have some time confusion. She sleeps all day, but when it's time for us to go to sleep, she becomes wide awake and stays that way through most of the night. What can we do to reverse this?*

A Many babies come into the world with their sleep-wake cycle established. In utero they wake up when Mom goes to sleep and go to sleep when Mom is active. You need to teach your infant that daytime is for feeding and interacting, and nighttime is for sleeping, not the reverse.

Here's how to get her on a normal sleep-wake cycle. During the day, wake your baby for feedings so that she does not sleep longer than three hours at a stretch. Play with her after each feeding for as long as she can stay awake and keep her with you in a stimulating environment. At night, keep your home calm and quiet—low lights, quiet music, soft voices, and minimal stimulation. When your baby awakens at night, respond to her quickly, but in a no-nonsense mode (keep talking to a minimum, and use a nightlight to see by). The message you want to communicate is that you expect your baby to fall back asleep. While you may have read that some babies can be put to sleep awake and will settle themselves off to sleep, it doesn't sound like your baby has this type of sleep temperament. She will need to be parented to sleep, not just put to sleep. This means she must be rocked and nursed.

In normal sleep development, you will find that as the months progress, your baby's stretches of daytime sleep will automatically shorten, while nighttime sleep will lengthen.

Cephalohematoma

Q *When our son was born, we noticed he had a lump on the back of his head. The doctor told us this was not abnormal, but we are getting worried. He is seven weeks old now and we can still feel the lump.*

A The lump you are feeling is called a cephalohematoma, which is caused by tiny blood vessels beneath the scalp breaking during delivery. This "goose egg" type of lump could take several months to disappear and may feel increasingly hard as the underlying blood calcifies. These lumps are harmless and happen in most babies during passage through the birth canal.

Because the lump is in the scalp and not actually in the brain, the bleeding will not bother your baby. Again, don't be alarmed if you still feel a slight lump a year later. If this were anything more than normal newborn scalp bleeding, your doctor would have informed you.

❧

Common Sense
on SIDS

Q *Reading the latest news about SIDS, I don't know whether to be excited or scared. If the Italian researchers are right, a newborn heart test may indicate whether my baby has a higher chance of dying from SIDS. What can you tell me about this new research? Should I have my baby tested? And what do I do if she's in the higher-risk group? I've also heard that putting her to sleep on her back will protect her. Is this true?*

A The Italian research you are speaking of was published in *The New England Journal of Medicine*. This study indicated that a specific abnormality in a newborn's electrocardiogram could be a sign that the child is at a higher-than-average risk for Sudden Infant Death Syndrome (SIDS). SIDS, which is also known as crib death, is the unexplained death of an infant under one year of age. It usually occurs between two and six months. It's important to note that even though SIDS is high on the list of parents' worries, it is uncommon, occurring in approximately one in one thousand infants. My concern about the screening test mentioned in the study is that it may cause unnecessary anxiety in parents. Also, this research is only a first study, and it needs to be confirmed by other investigations. In the long history of SIDS research, many studies have received a lot of publicity only to be disproven years later.

As the authors of the study suggested, electrocardiograph screening (a test that records the heart's electrical activity) could be effective on infants considered to be at high risk for SIDS. These include siblings of previous SIDS infants (although new insights show that these infants may not be at high risk), premature infants who have shown stop-breathing episodes (apnea) while being monitored, or infants of drug-abusing mothers. In the meantime, parents would be wise to take the following steps, which have been proven to lower the risk of SIDS:

- Put your baby to sleep on her back.
- Breastfeed your baby.
- Provide a safe sleeping environment, using a firm mattress and keeping the area free of plush toys or pillows.
- Don't smoke around your baby, before or after birth.

ℰ

A Newborn's Raised Soft Spot

Q *My baby is nine weeks old, and his soft spot still feels a little raised. Is this normal? He has a slight cold but no fever or any other signs of sickness.*

The soft spot, also called the fontanel, is an open area that provides room for an infant's growing brain. Located near the front of the head at the point where four major skull bones come together, the soft spot gradually becomes smaller until it closes by two years of age. While the area feels soft, it is actually covered by a thick, fibrous membrane, which isn't easily injured. Usually, the soft spot is flat or slightly raised. It is completely normal for the soft spot to be slightly raised, especially during the first nine months. Sometimes you can even see the soft spot pulsate.

It is difficult from your description to tell whether your baby's soft spot is a cause for concern. Run your hand over the top of his head; if you feel a distinct bump, call your doctor. There may be nothing wrong, but a bulging fontanel can signal internal pressure. If the area is not only bulging but also firm, your doctor may order an X ray called a CAT scan.

Sometimes a bulging fontanel is a sign of meningitis, but if your baby had this illness he would have other severe symptoms as well (such as a high fever, lethargy, and vomiting) that would have already prompted a visit to the doctor.

If the soft spot is sunken and accompanied by vomiting or diarrhea, abdominal pain, decreased urination, dry mouth, and no tears, you should call the doctor. Your baby could be suffering from dehydration.

⁂

Parenting a Detached Baby

Q *My eleven-week-old baby prefers sitting in a bouncer to being held, and she sleeps through the night in her crib rather than with me. Sometimes I feel my baby doesn't need me, although we both love nursing. I enjoyed co-sleeping*

*and using a sling with my other babies, and I miss that this
time around. Can I still have an attachment style of parenting with my baby?*

A Don't take your baby's detachment personally.
While most infants love to be held and cuddled, some
babies start off less cuddly and need time to warm up to
physical attachment. Some babies are just more comfortable being alone and need time to adjust to being touched.
If your baby sleeps through the night in her crib, that's
probably what's best for her, and there's no need to force
another sleeping arrangement on her. As long as your
daughter enjoys nursing, she probably gets all the holding
time she needs from this beautiful attachment relationship
with you.

Here are some ways you can help your baby grow
accustomed to the joys of physical touch:

- Gradually increase the amount of time you spend holding her each day.
- Try a daily infant massage, beginning with just a few
  minutes a day and easing into a twenty-minute ritual.
  For more information, we suggest the book *Infant Massage,* by Vimala Schneider McClure, or a video called
  Baby Massage, produced by Paccom Films (888-
  BABYTOUCH or 888-928-2466).
- Periodically try to carry her in a sling in the forward-
  facing position. This will help her feel less confined
  because she'll have a better view of what's going on.
  Your baby may find the snuggle hold or the cradle hold
  too confining.

❧

Baby Heartburn

Q *Our six-week-old son has terrible digestive problems and seems incredibly uncomfortable. Since he appeared a little gassy, we've been feeding him one to two drops of Mylicon daily, but ever since, he has been experiencing sporadic choking and even gasping within an hour after feeding. The choking appears out of nowhere and is sometimes preceded by vomiting, but his temperature remains normal. He also tends to cry for no apparent reason. Could he just be getting colicky?*

A   Most likely your son has a condition called gastroesophageal reflux (GER). The most common symptoms are spitting up shortly after a feeding, waking up at night in pain, colicky, painful episodes during the day, frequent coughs and colds, and general upset. With GER baby regurgitates irritating stomach acids into his esophagus—similar to what adults call heartburn.

As many as one-half of all babies are affected to some degree by reflux, and most of them do not need medication. Make an appointment with your doctor specifically for evaluation of GER. This can often be diagnosed by an X ray. If the X ray looks normal, your child could still have GER though, in which case your doctor will probably want to give your baby anti-reflux medication. These safe and effective medicines diminish the amount of acid in your baby's tummy and help it empty faster.

If your baby's GER doesn't require medication, here are some simple home remedies that you can use:

- Keep your baby upright for at least thirty minutes after each feeding.
- Offer smaller, more frequent feedings.
- Burp your baby well during and after each feeding.
- If you are using formula, experiment with different formulas, such as a soy formula or a hypoallergenic formula (Alimentum or Nutramigen). Allergy to formula can also contribute to your baby's symptoms.
- Elevate your baby's crib 30 degrees on one end. A reflux wedge, available at any infant-product store, will make this easier, or try Crib Blox, which fit under the legs of the crib.
- Wear your baby in a sling as much as possible to minimize crying (babies experience more reflux while crying). Several mothers in our practice have found that their infants' GER diminished after they wore them in a sling for several hours a day. The reason, they believe, is that babywearing after feeding promotes digestive organization. Gentle motion and closeness to mother seem to enhance intestinal function. Perhaps this is similar to the effect produced when a mother cat licks her kittens' abdomens after feeding.

One hidden cause of digestive problems in newborns is sensitivity to something in mother's milk (such as wheat or dairy) or an intolerance to formula. Breastfeeding moms can do a little detective work to try to figure out which foods need to be eliminated from their diet, starting with the most common culprits, which are dairy products. If after a week there is no improvement, other foods may have to be eliminated. Our book *The Fussy Baby Book* (Little, Brown, 1996) contains more detailed information about babies with digestive upsets or colic, including a step-by-step approach to diagnosis and treatment and how to eliminate foods from the mom's diet that upset baby's tummy.

The good news is that most babies outgrow GER by seven to eight months, mainly because they spend much of their day upright, taking advantage of gravity to hold food and milk in their stomach.

✍

Sharing Sleep with a GER Baby

Q *Our five-week-old son has been diagnosed with gastroesophageal reflux. He's been sleeping in our bed. Is there a way to safely continue this? The pediatrician suggested having our son sleep in a car seat. We are also worried about SIDS and the possible relationship with GER and stop-breathing episodes. We've been practicing attachment parenting and we'd rather not give up sleepsharing but want to do what's best for our baby.*

A Attachment parenting may lower the risk of SIDS and is beneficial for GER. So don't give up sleep-sharing. And we believe sleep-sharing lowers the risk of SIDS. The dilemma with SIDS and GER is that while sleeping on his back lowers a baby's risk of SIDS, it aggravates his GER. As a compromise, place your son to sleep on his left side facing you. In this position, gravity will help keep the milk down because the gastric inlet is higher than the outlet.

If your son has severe GER, try a reflux wedge (available at infant-product stores), which enables a baby to sleep propped up at a 30-degree angle. If the wedge is difficult to use in your bed, try it in a bedside co-sleeper (see Resources for Childcare Products and Information, page 129). The co-sleeper is an infant bed that attaches to your bed and gives baby his own sleeping space while keeping him within close touching and nursing distance.

Although back-sleeping is preferred to lower the risk of SIDS, the current recommendation is that babies with a medical condition that is improved by sleeping on their tummies should be placed to sleep on their tummies. GER is one of those conditions. In fact, GER itself can trigger stop-breathing episodes. As for your doctor's suggestion, a car seat is not advisable for sleeping because it bends a baby into a position that aggravates GER.

Although it tops parents' worry list, SIDS is actually rare (the current incidence is around one per one thousand babies). We advise you not to worry about SIDS and to place your baby to sleep in whatever position eases the discomfort of GER.

As your baby grows, his GER should diminish. In most cases GER subsides by the first birthday. For ways to lessen your son's discomfort in the meantime, see page 101.

⚮

Starting an Attachment Parenting Group

Q *We are starting an attachment-parenting group in a very conservative midwestern town. Do you have any suggestions on how to find speakers and potential members? Our La Leche League group is very small, and some of us do not belong to a church.*

A People have discovered how well attachment-parented children turn out, and we applaud your efforts! Giving infants attachment parenting during the formative first three years is one of the best investments you can make in your child, your family, and ultimately, your country. As a parent, you are raising someone else's future husband, wife, mother, or father. The style of parenting your child receives is the one he or she is likely to carry on into the next generation.

Attachment-parenting groups are forming all over the country. To form an attachment-parenting group, start with a nucleus of attachment parents. During your first meeting, discuss your goals and steps for growth. Each member should be encouraged to invite new parents to join the group.

When introducing attachment parenting to new parents, focus on the outcome rather than the method. Reassure skeptical moms and dads that this style of parenting increases their chances of raising well-disciplined, sensitive, joyful, and caring kids.

Begin with a discussion of the main baby B's:

• Birth
• Bonding
• Breastfeeding
• Babywearing
• Bed-sharing

Also talk about the need for parents to respond sensitively to their baby's cries and cues. Explain that these are just starter tips. Each parent can develop a parenting style that meets the needs of baby and the family's lifestyle.

It helps to market attachment parenting to expectant couples and new parents by focusing on what's in it for them in addition to the benefits for their baby. Admittedly, attachment parenting is not the easiest style of parenting. But while the first year may seem like one big give-a-thon, in reality the child is giving a lot back to the parents by teaching them to become expert cue readers. Explain how this style of parenting will make them experts on their baby. Attachment parenting builds trust that will enable them to discipline their baby intuitively and make baby more responsive to discipline. Above all, don't present it as a rigid set of rules that they must follow.

Stress that both parents and children can benefit even if they don't practice the complete attachment-parenting package. A mother who bottlefeeds can still become a sensitive attachment parent, and a dad who is unwilling to share his bed with his kids at night can practice some of the other attachment tips, such as wearing baby in a sling.

You'll find a lot of helpful information about starting and maintaining an attachment-parenting group by contacting Attachment Parenting International (see Resources for Childcare Products and Information, page 129).

For speakers, we suggest that you seek out local parents and pediatricians with personal and professional knowledge of attachment parenting.

$\mathcal{E}$

Cooling a Burning Bottom

Q *My daughter has diarrhea and a severe rash on her bottom. Our pediatrician suggested applying the antacid Maalox or Mylanta to her rear end for the acid burn. He said it would neutralize the acid that comes out in her diarrhea and irritates her skin. Is this okay to do, or is my doctor weird?*

A Where does a baby's rash come from? Start with ultrasensitive skin, add the chemicals in urine and stools, cover the area with a big "bandage," and rub it all together. Presto! You have diaper rash. If you keep this mixture together long enough, bacteria and fungi will begin to grow into the weakened skin, increasing the rash. Then, when the moist, fat folds rub together, the rash spreads to the creases of the groin.

What enters your baby's mouth further affects the skin on her rear end. Antibiotics, change of diet, and excess saliva during teething can all lead to diarrhea, which causes the acid burn on your baby's bottom. Since I have no personal experience using Maalox or Mylanta on babies' bottoms, let me suggest a more conventional treatment:

- Use ultra-absorbent diapers to keep your baby's skin as dry as possible.
- Rinse baby's bottom after every diaper change. Sensitive skin does best with plain water, although some bottoms need a mild soap. Sore bottoms may react to the chemicals in disposable baby wipes—especially those containing alcohol.
- Dip baby's bottom in a baking soda bath (add ¼ cup of baking soda to her bath water) to neutralize the acid.
- Blot the skin dry with a soft towel and avoid excessive rubbing or scrubbing with a strong soap on irritated skin. One of our babies had such sensitive skin that even towel blotting reddened it. Instead, we used a hair dryer (held 12 inches away on the lowest setting) to blow-dry her bottom.
- Keep bottoms up. Expose baby's bottom to the air while she is sleeping and occasionally to a ten-minute ray of sunlight through a closed window.
- Apply a lubricant, such as Soothe and Heal with Lansinoh, as a barrier cream.

Diaper rash is an unfortunate fact of life for bottom-covered babies. But like all the other nuisance stages of infancy, it too will pass.

ℒ&

Babies and Breath-Holding

Q *When our two-month-old is crying hard, she sometimes starts to hyperventilate, turns bright red, then holds her breath. Finally she takes a deep breath and falls asleep in exhaustion. Is it normal for babies to hold their breath? My friends' babies don't do this, and it's scary.*

A While upsetting to parents, breath-holding is rarely a cause for concern. These episodes, almost always triggered by a crying jag, are usually over quickly. A baby cries harder and harder, starts to hyperventilate, then stops breathing. Just as her parents are ready to panic, baby takes a deep breath, the color returns to her face, and all is well.

Breath-holding is most common between six months and two to three years, though it can begin earlier and run later. Spells usually subside when a child is old enough to express her feelings in words. Breath-holding is often brought on by anger, frustration, pain, overtiredness, or overstimulation. Most incidents are linked to temper tantrums, though it's unlikely that this is the case with a newborn.

The best way to handle breath-holding is to stay calm. If your baby senses that you are tense, she may become even more upset. Reassure her that everything's okay by holding and calming her.

To cut down on breath-holding episodes, keep a diary to pinpoint events that cause them. Do they usually happen at the end of the day, when your baby is tired? Do they occur on days when she's had a lot of visitors? Are they linked to particularly fussy days? When these situations occur again, intervene with calming words and gestures or distracting activities.

Getting Baby to Take a Bottle

Q *I've breastfed my eight-week-old daughter since birth, supplementing only when I need to be away for a short period of time. My baby prefers the breast and has a difficult time taking the bottle. We've tried various nipples, including a nurser that claims to be like a human nipple. She won't even take a pacifier. I have to return to work soon, so any suggestions would be appreciated.*

A   Your daughter has gourmet tastes and has been dining first-class since birth. It's unlikely that she will willingly accept less palatable cuisine (formula) and a bland restaurant (the bottle) at the same time.

We suggest putting your pumped breast milk in a bottle. Then have someone else—your husband or substitute caregiver—give her the bottle when you can't breastfeed. Many breastfed infants will not take a bottle from their mother. After all, they associate Mom with breastfeeding, and it confuses them. If you're unable to pump enough milk (try a Medela double-pumping system), gradually get your infant used to formula by adding increasing amounts of formula to the pumped breast milk.

You mentioned trying a nurser that is like a human nipple. Actually, there's no such thing. The art of juggling bottle- and breastfeeding is to choose a nipple that requires your baby to open her mouth wide while bottlefeeding, as she does on your areola while breastfeeding. With some nursers, babies tend to suck only on the nubbin of the nipple and don't exert enough sucking pressure to draw out the wider part of the nipple (as the manufacturer claims). A baby who gets used to sucking on the nubbin of an artificial nipple may get in the habit of breastfeeding that way, giving Mom an uncomfortable case of sore nipples.

Try Nuk or Evenflo nipples. These have a wider base. Ask your caregiver to make sure your baby opens her mouth enough to suck on the wide base of the nipple, not just on the tip. Breastfeed before you leave for work in the morning, and ask your caregiver not to feed your baby for at least an hour before you are due home from work. As soon as you return, enjoy happy-to-see-you breastfeeding time with your baby.

Point out to your caregiver that feeding is a social interaction, not just a way of delivering milk. During bottle-feeding, your caregiver should hold your baby in the same position you do while breastfeeding and offer lots of eye-to-eye contact and caressing. Some very selective gourmets hold out for Mom to return from work and refuse to take a bottle. If your baby is still holding out by four months of age, try introducing solid foods (mashed bananas, rice cereal, and pears), which your caregiver can feed her during the day. Then you can nurse as soon as you get home.

A perk for continuing to breastfeed after going back to work is that not only are you continuing to provide your baby with optimal nutrition, but breastfeeding releases relaxing hormones in your body, which help you unwind after a tense day at work. On weekends and holidays, resume full-time breastfeeding.

✍

Accommodating Your Baby's Need Level

Q *My ten-week-old baby recently began full-time day care. Things were fine when he attended day care part-time, but now he cries constantly. The staff is worried about him—although when I pick him up at the end of the day, he's a perfect angel. I've sent my pillowcase to day care with him, hoping to quell his separation anxiety. I also plan to make a tape recording of my voice. Do you have any other suggestions? Should I spend my lunch break with him? He also sleeps with me—should I stop that? How long will this last?*

A Choosing substitute care for your tiny baby is one of the most crucial decisions you will ever make. This is the time in your child's life when he forms deep and lasting impressions about the caregiving world, and you want him to perceive that world as a warm and trusting place. To encourage this perception, it's important to choose a caregiver who shares your parenting philosophy. Avoid caregivers who believe in letting babies cry it out. This mind-set will only increase your baby's protests and separation anxiety or—worse—induce apathy and cause your baby to resign himself to a lower level of care and trust than he truly needs.

Sending your pillowcase and tape recordings of your voice to day care with your baby are excellent ways to help him feel connected to you while you're apart. We do recommend that you spend time with your baby during the lunch hour and that you continue sleeping with him at night. In fact, sharing sleep is becoming a much more common infant-care practice. Many mothers find sleep-sharing beneficial because it allows them to reconnect with their babies at night to make up for the time apart during the day. We strongly recommend that you get your baby used to being worn in a sling as much as possible and that you teach your caregiver to do this as well. Studies show that babies who are carried at least several hours a day cry a lot less than those who are not, so insist on this level of attention from your baby's caregiver. If your baby's crying persists, have him checked out by your pediatrician.

When making decisions about your parenting style, try to see things from your baby's perspective. You may be blessed with a high-need baby who has high expectations and needs in order to thrive physically, emotionally, and intellectually and a strong personality to assert that his needs are met.

One of the most important things we've learned is to be aware of each child's unique need level. Every baby is born with a certain level of need, and most babies are able to communicate to their caregivers what they need. For example, a baby who cries when put down but settles happily in someone's arms has a high need to be held in order to thrive. This need-level concept is beneficial for both babies and caregivers. What creates problems is when parents and caregivers try to force a style of care onto an infant that doesn't match her level of need. A high-need baby can bring out the best and worst in a caregiver, but caregivers who respond sensitively to a baby's needs develop a higher level of giving and develop strategies and techniques for baby comforting that they may not have had with a lesser-need child. That is why the term "demanding" should be considered a positive character trait—at least in the first six months of life.

Above all, let your intuition guide you on whether you have found the right caregiver-baby match. When in doubt, change caregivers or juggle your working hours if you can. A high-need baby may temporarily derail a mother's career plans and cause her to take a different track. But choosing another track often ends up benefiting both mother and baby. Examine your options: Can you work part-time or job-share? Is flextime an option for you? Can you work for a company with infant-care facilities on-site? Can you negotiate a couple of extra months of maternity leave with your employer and work from home? In our practice, we've written many "prescriptions" for mothers to present to their employers supporting their need to make a change in their job situation.

Juggling work and parenting to meet the needs of your entire family is one of the most challenging tasks you'll ever face. It's important to remember, however, that babyhood lasts for a very short time. This precious time in your child's life is a tape that cannot be rewound.

✍

Traveling Overseas with Baby

Q *My husband and I are planning a trip to Chile when our son is between two and three months old. What are the health risks for a child this age traveling overseas?*

A   Every country has different health risks and conse-
quent recommendations, and they often change from
month to month. For the most up-to-date information, you
should call the Centers for Disease Control's International
Travelers' Hotline at 877-FYI-TRIP or go to their Web site
at www.cdc.gov and look for travelers' health information.
In addition, I recommend drinking bottled water rather
than tap water in any foreign country you are visiting.

Foreign diseases aren't the only factor to consider when
you travel. To make any plane trip (foreign or domestic)
safer and more comfortable for the whole family, consider
the following:

- If your baby's not used to being carried in a sling or
  other carrier, start using one now. These useful devices
  enable you to carry a small child through busy airports
  and crowds with minimal exposure to strangers.
- Book a no-smoking flight. There are still some international airlines that allow smoking. Tiny air passages are
  particularly sensitive to air pollution from cigarette
  smoke. Even if you're seated in the so-called no-smoking section of an aircraft, you're still going to inhale pol-
  lutants from the smoking section. (Think of it as trying
  to chlorinate half a swimming pool—it can't be done.)
- Nurse your baby or give him a bottle while the plane is
  ascending. Tiny ears are particularly sensitive to changes
  in altitude, and sucking on something will help prevent
  uncomfortable pressure from building up in his eustachian tubes. You might also consider waking your little one
  for a feeding when the plane begins to descend, since
  eustachian tubes don't adjust well to altitude changes
  while a baby's sleeping and may therefore cause him
  discomfort.

- Give your baby extra fluids to drink, since babies, like adults, can get dehydrated easily on long flights.
- Spritz your baby's nose with a saline nasal spray every few hours. The low humidity of cabin air is likely to make his tiny nose stuff up, so he'll appreciate the relief these sprays bring. (Look for them in small over-the-counter squirt bottles at your local pharmacy.)
- Request a bulkhead seat. In many cases, these seats are equipped with pull-down bassinets and have extra floor space.

✍

Colic Means Baby Is Hurting

Q *My three-month-old baby girl was born ten weeks early. I stopped breastfeeding at seven weeks and have been giving her formula. She began eating a lot (6 to 9 ounces at each feeding) and became constipated. My pediatrician suggested that I stop feeding her so much, but now my baby has colic. Although she has no temperature, she is sleeping more than usual. Today she woke up with a hoarse cry. Is this normal for colicky babies because they scream so much?*

A Here's a trade secret we've learned from more than twenty-five years practicing pediatrics: Colic is a five-letter word that means "the doctor doesn't know." In our view, it's too easy to tag a baby as colicky and quickly dismiss the problem. We prefer the phrase "hurting baby" to "colicky baby."

Colic can stem from a variety of causes. Your baby may hurt because she is allergic to the formula. In fact, anytime you see a change in behavior or bowel habits following a change in feeding, it's reasonable to suspect that the food and the intestines don't agree with one another. Gastro-esophageal reflux (GER) is another hidden cause of colicky behavior. As in the case of adult heartburn, your baby regurgitates stomach acids up into her esophagus, causing a painful sensation shortly after feeding.

To make feeding less hurtful and more pleasant for your baby, try changing formulas. Milk-based formulas are most likely the cause of her discomfort because of an allergy to the protein in milk. Try switching to a soy-based formula. But before making the switch, jot down your baby's usual symptoms so that you can objectively record any changes. If you notice no improvement after a week on soy formula, try a hypoallergenic formula, such as Alimentum, Nutramigen, or Pregestimil. In these protein-hydrolysate formulas, the potentially allergenic proteins have been predigested, so they're easier on baby's digestive system.

Also, try smaller, more frequent feedings. Some babies, while not allergic to formula itself, simply can't digest too much at one feeding. But overfeeding is probably not the cause of your baby's constipation. It is more likely to cause diarrhea than constipation. Constipation does, however, frequently present as colic. Give your baby an extra 8 ounces of water each day and experiment with formulas that are less constipating. If she strains to have a bowel movement, insert half of an infant glycerin suppository into her rectum to help her go.

The fact that your baby seems to be sleeping more than usual makes us doubt that a formula allergy or GER is at the root of her discomfort. Babies with intestinal upset usually sleep less and wake up frequently with painful cries. Crying accompanied by more sleeping suggests an emotional reason for your baby's discomfort more than a dietary or medical one—though babies can hurt so much for medical reasons that they sleep more simply out of exhaustion from crying. Has there been a recent change in caregivers, sleeping arrangements, or the family's lifestyle? If you have recently returned to work, try carrying her in a sling as much as you can on your days off to see if this settles her crying.

Your baby's hoarseness may be caused by her excessive crying. But it's unusual even for colicky babies to be hoarse. The fact that your little one is crying herself hoarse is all the more reason to get to the bottom of why she is hurting. Keep working to identify any dietary or caregiver changes until you are able to ease your baby's discomfort. Colicky behavior that continues beyond six months strongly suggests an underlying medical cause, but the good news is that even unexplained colic usually passes by six months.

҈

Calming a Tense Baby

Q *Even when I try to comfort my baby, she seems so uncomfortable and cries aloud. My pediatrician said she has colic and should outgrow this, but can't I help her relax in the meantime?*

A Try these four time-tested holds for relaxing a tense baby in your arms:

1. The arm drape (also called the "football hold"). Rest baby's head in the crook of your elbow, drape baby's stomach along your forearm, and grasp the diaper area firmly. Your forearm will press against baby's tense abdomen.

2. The colic curl. Babies who tense their tummy and arch their back often settle in this position. Slide baby's back down your chest, and encircle your arms under his bottom. Curl baby up, with his head facing forward and his back resting against your chest. As a gas reliever, pump baby's thighs in a bicycling motion.

3. The handstand (beginning around age four months). Let baby face forward with his back up against your chest as he stands on one of your hands. Lean slightly back to discourage baby from lunging forward, and be ready to catch the lunger with the other hand in case he does. (Press your other hand up against baby's abdomen if that warm pressure seems to help.)

4. The neck nestle. Here's a high-touch baby-calmer where Dad shines. While walking, dancing, or lying with your baby on your chest, snuggle her head against the front of your neck, and drape your chin over baby's head. Then hum or sing a low-pitched melody like "Ol' Man River" while swaying from side to side. The vibration of your larynx and jaw against your baby's sensitive skull can often lull the tense baby right to sleep. Some of my most memorable moments as the father of infants are of holding my babies in the neck nestle position while singing the Sears family "Go to Sleep" song:

> *Go to sleep, go to sleep,*
> *Go to sleep my little baby.*
> *Go to sleep, go to sleep,*
> *Go to sleep my little girl.*

For added comforting and sleep-inducing success, try the above holds while walking or dancing with your baby. Add moving attractions, such as waves on the beach or moving traffic.

Along with motion, most babies are soothed by sounds, preferably ones that remind them of the womb. The most calming sounds are rhythmic, monotonous, low-pitched, and humming in quality, with slowly rising and falling crescendos and decrescendos, and a pattern that repeats at a rate of sixty to seventy pulses per minute. Infant-product manufacturers have capitalized on research into soothing sounds by producing a variety of sleep-inducing sound makers that use white noise—a monotonous, repetitive sound involving a wide range of frequencies audible to the human ear; this will lull an overloaded mind into sleep. However, you don't need to go out and buy a special tape or gadget to lull your baby to sleep.

Sights That Distract

Q *Sometimes my baby daughter cries and gets wrapped up in her own cries. I try to distract her and that works sometimes. Do you have any suggestions for ways to stop a crying fit?*

A A captivating image can distract some babies in the midst of a crying fit and sidetrack others before they have a chance to howl. Try these sights to help your tearful newborn:

- *Magic mirror.* Hold the fussy baby in front of a mirror and let her watch her own drama. Place her hand or bare foot against its image on the mirror's surface, and watch the intrigued baby grow silent.

- *Happy face.* Spend a lot of time in face-to-face contact with your baby, showing baby exaggerated (but pleasant) facial expressions. Remember which facial expressions he likes, and replay them later when he fusses. High-need babies demand a lot of connecting experiences, and face-to-face, eye-to-eye contact is what they need in order to know they are being heard and seen clearly. All this connecting is why high-need babies grow up to be such good communicators, sensitive to the body language and nonverbal cues of others. They get plenty of practice.

- *Silly face.* Give baby a sudden change of face. Put on your silliest or most dramatic facial gestures and direct them at baby. These antics take most babies by surprise, causing them to forget (at least temporarily) why they are fussing.

✍

Healing Tenseness

Q *My baby is definitely a high-need baby and must touch me or my husband twenty-four hours a day. I understand all about attachment parenting, but sometimes I get tired of being the "body on call." Is this constant touch vital?*

A   Every baby needs a great deal of touching. High-need babies need more (of course!). This is because high-need babies have tense muscles that need help relaxing.

Infant massage is an enjoyable way to touch and soothe your infant. You can learn the art of infant massage from an infant massage instructor (ask your local childbirth instructor if she can recommend someone).

Try these Sears favorites for relaxing your high-need baby:

- *The warm fuzzy.* Here's a high-touch soother where father can really shine. Dads, lie down and drape baby skin-to-skin over your chest, placing baby's ear over your heart. As baby senses the rhythm of your heartbeat plus the up-and-down motion of your breathing, you will feel the tense baby relax. His fists will uncurl and his limbs will dangle limply over your chest.
- *Nestle nursing.* Undress your baby down to a diaper and lie down on the bed together. Curl up womblike around your baby, face-to-face, tummy-to-tummy, and let baby nurse. This is especially nice if Mom's clothing allows for lots of skin contact. The natural calm that comes from being touched, from sucking, and from feeling your breathing and heartbeat along with gentle strokes from your fingers will relax even the fussiest baby and send her off into peaceful sleep. Martha calls this hold the "teddy bear snuggle."
- *A shared warm bath.* Mothers of high-need babies have put in many hours of hydrotherapy because it works! Recline in a half-full tub, and have Dad hand baby to you. If you are alone, have baby "stand by" in an infant seat right next to the tub until you are ready to bring her

into the tub. Place baby tummy-to-tummy against your chest, and let her breastfeed in the water (your nipples being a couple of inches above the surface). Baby will float a bit while nursing, which adds to the soothing effect. Taking a bath with baby helps relax Mom as well. Leave the faucet running a bit and the tub's drain open. The flow of the warm water not only provides a sooth-ing sound but also keeps the water comfortably warm.

❧

A Preference for Pacifiers

Q   *Help! My twelve-week-old son has suddenly become dependent on his pacifier. Before, we used it only in the car when I was unable to comfort him physically. Now he gives hunger cues but becomes hysterical when I try to nurse him. When I finally give him his pacifier in desperation, he makes loud moaning noises until he falls asleep. I don't know if this is related, but he also has started going five to six hours between feedings during the day. He seems healthy and doesn't look dehydrated, but I'm concerned.*

A   Infants are born with an intense need to suck, and sometimes they go through a stage where their sucking need intensifies. It can be even more frustrating when, for unexplained reasons, your baby prefers a pacifier to you. Here's how to decrease your little one's dependence on the pacifier and woo him back to the breast:

- *Feed him more frequently.* Going five to six hours between feedings during the day is unlikely to meet your baby's sucking needs or deliver enough nutrition.

- *Eliminate distractions during nursing.* At this age, your infant's more acute visual development makes him easily distracted during nursing. He may become "Mr. Suck-a-Little-Look-a-Little." At feeding time, take him into a quiet room and get down to the business of nursing.

- *Establish a routine.* A daily nap-nursing routine has worked for our family. At least twice a day, lie down with your baby and nap-nurse—much as you did when he was a newborn. This peaceful reconnection in a quiet room is likely to bring him back to the breast.

- *Offer your finger.* Periodically let your baby suck on your finger instead of the pacifier—even during the nap-nursing time—if he doesn't want to feed.

- *Try nursing on the move.* When one of our babies went through a similar nursing quirk, Martha wore him around the house in a sling and nursed him frequently while she tended to other things.

⌇

Causes of Diarrhea

Q *Our three-month-old daughter has had diarrhea for over ten days. I was breastfeeding her exclusively at first, but during the last few weeks we've given her some bottled milk because my milk supply has dropped. Her stools are still green in color. Other than that, my baby has no fever or any other symptoms of illness. Could her diarrhea be caused by something I'm eating?*

A Your baby's diarrhea is most likely due to an intestinal infection. As long as she does not have a fever, abdominal pain, or increasing weight loss, there is no need to worry.

Two types of germs cause diarrhea in infants: viruses and bacteria. Viral infections are usually more of a nuisance type of diarrhea in an otherwise well baby and heal themselves without treatment. Bacterial infections are usually associated with fever, abdominal pain, and increasing weight loss, and may need an antibiotic. Let the old saying "No weight loss, no problem" be your guide. If your baby isn't losing weight and isn't particularly bothered by the diarrhea, it will probably go away without treatment.

Keep in mind, however, that the intestines are slow to heal; it could take six to eight weeks for your baby's bowel movements to return to normal consistency. Breast milk helps the intestines heal and is best tolerated by an irritated intestinal lining. Cow's milk, on the other hand, may aggravate the diarrhea. Try nursing your baby more often to increase your milk supply. If she needs a supplement, a soy-based formula would be more intestines friendly. Your main goal in treating diarrhea is to prevent your baby from getting dehydrated (weight loss is a sign of dehydration). To provide additional fluids, feed her 2 ounces of diluted white grape juice several times a day. Unlike other fruit juices that may worsen diarrhea, white grape juice contains the type of sugar that makes it easy on the intestines.

♋

Simple Joys for a Gifted Baby

Q *Although my son is only three months old, he can find his mouth, feet, penis, and even his pacifier when he drops it. I would be very interested in what you think. If you think he is gifted, please tell me what I can do to help further his development.*

A Obviously you have a gifted child who is off the charts in the area of motor development. But don't feel it is your immediate responsibility to stimulate him. "Infant stim" has become a buzzword in psychological circles, causing parents to feel they owe their child constant stimulation—sort of like a hot meal and a warm winter jacket. There is no evidence that fancy toys make brighter babies. When evaluating the influence of toys and programs versus individuals on infant development, parents still emerge as the most important factor.

We believe that everything you do with your baby is infant stimulation. One of the most natural stimulators is wearing your baby in a sling around the house and outside. Being in your arms allows your baby to view his environment at a more meaningful level. And being outside provides many moving attractions for babies, such as traffic, limbs and leaves on trees, and children frolicking in a playground. So don't feel that because your baby is gifted he needs more stuff. The right stuff for your little one is parent-infant interaction on a daily basis. For now just have fun with your baby and enjoy his individual development.

Hand toys are the most appropriate at this age. The simplest and most educational (and inexpensive) toy for a three- or four-month-old is a red rubber ring 3 to 4 inches in diameter. A baby can control this all-purpose object completely. He holds it in one hand, brings it to his midline, grabs it with his other hand, pulls on it with both hands, and releases it with one hand while holding on with the other. All the time, he follows it with his eyes and gums it when it finds its inevitable destination (his mouth).

Babies get bored with the same old toy. The human face (yours!) is an excellent stimulus for babies. It reacts to what baby is doing, and it's constantly changing. The best way to approach a baby is to follow the look-talk-touch sequence. First, establish eye contact with the baby, then talk to him, and finally pick him up for play. Avoid bombardment. Babies have short attention spans—only four to ten seconds. Short, frequent playful interactions are more meaningful than longer, forced ones. When you're interacting with your baby, watch for "stop signs." Just as babies signal when they're ready for interaction (with smiles, eye contact, or hands-out gesturing), they also let you know when they want to stop (vacant staring, turning away, or a furrowed brow). Many fathers take longer than mothers to recognize these signals. Because dads are seldom allowed the luxury of long periods of unscheduled time with their infants, they tend to rush to initiate a playful interaction and can end up overstimulating their baby.

Resources for Childcare Products and Information

Parenting and Pediatric Information

www.parenting.com. An informative Web site on parenting issues. Dr. Bill and Martha Sears answer parenting questions and host frequent chats and workshops.
www.askdrsears.com. A comprehensive Web site on healthcare information for infants and children.

Baby Carriers

A soft baby carrier is one of the most useful parenting products you and your baby will enjoy. Consult the following resources for information on sling-type carriers and step-by-step instructions on using a sling.

The Original BabySling
800-421-0526 or www.originalbabysling.com or
www.nojo.com

Crown Crafts Infant Products
310-763-8100 or www.crowncraftsinfantproducts.com

www.AskDrSears.com   Visit our store.

Bedside Co-Sleepers

A bedside co-sleeper lets baby and parents sleep close to one another yet still have their own space. This criblike bed safely attaches to the parents' bed.

Arm's Reach Co-Sleeper
800-954-9353 or 818-879-9353 or www.armsreach.com

Nursing Clothing and Accessories

Motherwear   800-950-2500 or www.motherwear.com

Breastfeeding Help and Resources

La Leche League International (LLLI)
800-435-8316 or 847-519-7730 or
www.lalecheleague.org

**International Lactation Consultant Association
(ILCA)** 919-787-5181 or www.ilca.org

Corporate Lactation Program by Medela
800-435-8316 or www.medela.com

Attachment Parenting International
615-298-4334 or www.attachmentparenting.org

Mothering Multiples

National Organization of Mothers of Twins Clubs, Inc.
877-540-2200 or 615-595-0936 or www.nomotc.org

Index

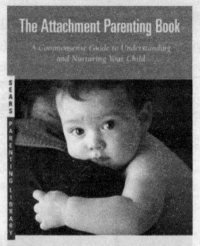

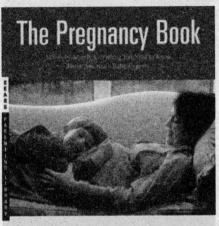

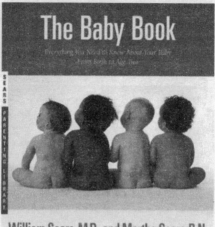